Praise for Dr. Shawn

The Natural Vet's Guide ~~to Preventing~~
and Treating Cancer in Dogs

"An eminently qualified veterinarian who has contributed to *Dog Fancy* and other publications, Messonnier is here to help. With a passion for alternative treatments, he offers this comprehensive and current work.... He presents clear and understandable information for lay readers, decoding often confusing medical jargon.... Messonnier's newest work is exceptionally well done and comes highly recommended."

— *Library Journal*

"Dr. Messonnier provides readers — both veterinarians and pet owners — with an understandable overview of the latest research on preventing and treating cancer as well as when and how natural medicine does and, more important, does not play a role. The book also offers sound advice and clear directions for pet owners who are interested in the complementary approach.... It is a welcome addition to the veterinary literature."

— *Veterinary Forum*

"Dr. Messonnier presents cancer treatment options for dogs, utilizing the latest research. Additionally, he writes about a slew of holistic prevention options — such as acupuncture, chiropractic, homeopathy, nutritional supplements, and herbal remedies — and discusses how to use these therapies as complementary treatments for dogs that have already been diagnosed with cancer."

— *Tails* pet magazines

"This is a book for every dog/human companion home.... [It] offers the kind of reference and medical information applicable to the overall health and well-being of any dog. Please own it, and share it, especially with your veterinarian."

— *Lajoie*

"Dr. Messonnier's landmark work is a comprehensive, practical guide to a subject that every pet owner should be concerned about."

— Michael T. Murray, ND, coauthor of
How to Prevent and Treat Cancer with Natural Medicine

"This is a truly important book, vital to all dog owners. Cancer is a leading cause of death in older dogs, and unfortunately, veterinarians are seeing cancer in younger and younger animals as well. As they say, an ounce of prevention is worth a pound of cure, but with this book, you get a ton of each! This is, without question, the most comprehensive book available on this topic."

— Jean Hofve, DVM, holistic feline veterinarian and
founder of Littlebigcat.com

"This responsible and wonderful contribution is clear and pragmatic. Dr. Shawn Messonnier provides a better understanding of canine cancer and the best treatments that combine conventional and complementary methods. Readers will obtain not only a better appreciation of the author's expertise on the subject but also his compassion for his canine patients and their owners. A must-read for those interested in proactive and preventive measures against this disease."

— Thomas Nelson, president of the Perseus Foundation,
a nonprofit organization dedicated to
animal cancer research and education

THE NATURAL VET'S GUIDE *to*

PREVENTING and TREATING ARTHRITIS IN DOGS and CATS

THE NATURAL VET'S GUIDE *to*

PREVENTING and TREATING ARTHRITIS IN DOGS and CATS

SHAWN MESSONNIER, DVM

SECOND EDITION

New World Library
Novato, California

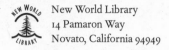
New World Library
14 Pamaron Way
Novato, California 94949

Text design by Tona Pearce Myers

4646 4102 7/11

Library of Congress Cataloging-in-Publication Data
Messonnier, Shawn.
  The natural vet's guide to preventing and treating arthritis in dogs and cats / Shawn Messonnier.
    p.   cm.
Rev. ed. of: Arthritis solution for dogs / Shawn Messonnier, © 2000.
Includes bibliographical references and index.
ISBN 978-1-57731-975-7 (pbk.)
  1. Dogs—Diseases. 2. Arthritis in animals. I. Messonnier, Shawn. Arthritis solution for dogs. II. Title.
SF992.A77M47 2011
636.089'6722—dc22   2011009509

First printing, June 2011
ISBN 978-1-57731-975-7
Printed in Canada on 100% postconsumer-waste recycled paper

New World Library is a proud member of the Green Press Initiative.

10 9 8 7 6 5 4 3 2 1

CONTENTS

PREFACE

ARTHRITIS IS A COMMON MEDICAL PROBLEM in dogs and cats. Many useful integrative, or natural, therapies exist for the arthritic pet, including antioxidants, herbal preparations, homeopathic remedies, magnetic therapy, raw food and glandular supplements, chiropractic, massage, laser, homotoxicology, and acupuncture. Which therapy or therapies will most help your pet depends on a number of factors and should be determined after careful consultation with your holistic veterinarian.

Throughout this book, I have tried to present information in a truly holistic fashion, remaining as objective as possible. Of course, I am biased toward the therapies I use frequently and the products I have personally tested and proven to be safe and effective. When possible in the book, I have indicated this bias.

For some therapies, there exists a large body of well-designed, scientifically coordinated research studies. For other therapies, doctors do not have controlled studies but instead rely on clinical experience (we know these therapies work because we've used them for many years and have seen positive effects). Still other therapies show promise in people, and although their effectiveness in pets is unknown, they may be useful.

My hope is that you and your doctor will find a natural therapy that helps your arthritic pet and reduces the need for medical therapies that are potentially more harmful. Each pet is an individual and must be treated as such, and what works for one pet may not be helpful for another. I am confident that, with the large number of natural therapies available, you will find one that helps your dog or cat and allows you to either reduce the amount of medication needed to keep your pet comfortable or eliminate medication altogether.

Information is always changing, and new treatments are popping up as I write this book. Future editions will update you on important and promising new therapies.

I would appreciate hearing from you about how I can improve future editions so that we can make the world a healthier, more holistic place for our pets!

ABOUT NATURAL
SUPPLEMENTS

IN THIS BOOK, I mention many natural supplements that can assist pets that have arthritis. I have attempted to be as objective as possible and to refrain from promoting any particular products. Still every doctor has favorites that have worked best in his or her practice, and I have pointed out my favorites when necessary. Since there are many products available to help your pet, I encourage you to work with your doctor to find the ones most suitable for your pet.

The information in this book is not meant to be a substitute for medical advice. Natural therapies are not necessarily safe and may interact negatively with other therapies, including conventional medical therapies, and this can result in harm to your pet. Before beginning any of the therapies discussed in this book, you should consult with a licensed veterinarian who is trained in the use of natural therapies.

A NOTE *about* CATS

ONE OF MY FAVORITE SAYINGS IS: "Cats are not small dogs." We can't treat cats like small dogs, and so treating a cat with arthritis, while similar to treating an arthritic dog, is somewhat different. Generally, in this book what I say about dogs also applies to cats, except where I specifically indicate otherwise.

Although we try to avoid the unnecessary use of medications such as nonsteroidal anti-inflammatory drugs (NSAIDs) in both dogs and cats, these drugs can be used safely to relieve pain and inflammation in cats when absolutely necessary. But with cats, we must be much more careful when using such drugs. Because of a deficiency in liver enzymes, cats are not able to adequately metabolize and detoxify many medications, including NSAIDs. Practically, this means certain drugs that can be safely administered to dogs can easily become toxic or even fatal when administered to cats at the same dosage or while using the same dosing regimen. And fewer NSAIDs are approved for use in cats. When necessary, these drugs can be used in cats at a different dosage and with a different dosing regimen (usually a few times per week in cats, rather than a few times per day as in dogs).

In general, joint supplements safe for dogs can be used in cats. There are exceptions, and it is important to work with your veterinarian to identify the supplements that could be toxic to your cat and to avoid those.

While acupuncture, chiropractic, laser therapy, and physical therapy can all be performed safely on cats, felines often are not the easiest patients to treat. The use of these therapies, then, is not as common for cats as for dogs but can be helpful if the patient is cooperative.

Because it can be difficult to administer oral products to cats, some may require conventional medications in addition to oral supplements, herbs, or homeopathics. Alternatively, cats that refuse oral natural therapies may be easier to treat with physical therapies, such as laser therapy.

Cats are as likely as dogs to get arthritis. Middle-aged and older cats that seem to have slowed down, refuse to jump up onto furniture, stop using the litter box, or act old and cranky may be suffering from arthritis (or other problems, especially dental disease, so be sure to get your cat checked by your veterinarian if you see any of these signs).

Fortunately, when properly diagnosed and treated, cats respond as well to natural therapies (and conventional medications when needed) as do their arthritic canine counterparts.

UNDERSTANDING *the* HOLISTIC APPROACH *to* TREATING ARTHRITIS

MY WEDNESDAY MORNING BEGAN with one of my favorite pets, Jake, a ten-year-old Labrador retriever. On this morning, his owner shared with me that Jake seemed to be having more difficulty getting around. This is a common complaint from owners of older large-breed dogs. Many of these pets do exhibit varying degrees of lameness as they age. Many times the cause is something simple, such as hip dysplasia or arthritis. Other times the culprit is something more sinister, such as cancer or degeneration of the spinal nerves.

In order to determine the cause of Jake's lameness, we sedated him and took radiographs (X-rays) of his hips and spine. In Jake's case, these simple radiographs showed mild hip dysplasia with secondary arthritis. Because Jake's owner was holistic-minded and preferred natural therapies over medications when possible, I started Jake on a regimen of fatty acids and nutritional supplements. Within a few weeks, he was moving around much better, and he would never experience any of the side effects that can be seen in pets that are prescribed chronic therapy with anti-arthritic medications.

Lameness is a common symptom of arthritis in older dogs. Interestingly, we are seeing more arthritis in older cats as well. Although younger dogs and cats, too, can become lame from a variety of causes, as is the case in people, the joints of our aging pets begin to show the wear and tear of activity that has occurred over a number of years. Many older dogs and cats live with joint instability — specifically caused by hip dysplasia or spinal problems — for years, often without the owner even knowing the pet has any underlying problems.

Because lameness caused by arthritis is common in the geriatric pet, and because many doctors are not comfortable treating geriatric pets, older dogs and cats are often ignored or improperly treated. Instead of performing diagnostic tests to determine the cause and severity of the problem, and instead of searching for the least harmful treatment options, many doctors just try to make such a pet comfortable for whatever time it has left. While there is nothing wrong with making pets comfortable, there is no reason to think that a geriatric pet with arthritis is on its last legs. Many older arthritic pets can still have months if not years of good-quality living if doctors treat them as they would younger pets. There's no reason for doctors to reach for the "magic shot" of corticosteroids, or other potentially harmful medications, such as nonsteroidal anti-inflammatory medications, if other, more natural, safer alternatives are available.

In this book, I discuss the most common treatment options available for arthritic dogs and cats. By wisely combining conventional and alternative treatment options, veterinarians can properly diagnose the lame pet's problems and attempt to ease its discomfort without cutting short its life.

> *The doctor's primary responsibility is to take care of his or her patients.*

When it comes to treating the arthritic pet, owners have many options. The reason for the large number of options is that there is truly no one "best" treatment for every pet. I hold the holistic belief that each pet is an individual and must be treated as such. I discuss this philosophy with owners right from the start. What worked for the last arthritic dog or cat I treated may not work for their pets. Additionally, each owner is different and has different wants and a different budget. Some owners want to do everything possible for their pets. Money is not an object, and they often allow us to experiment with quite a number of unique treatments. Others opt for a bit less and may not mind letting their pets take medications such as corticosteroids or nonsteroidal anti-inflammatory drugs (NSAIDs) for the long haul. Still others want no medications at all and opt for more natural therapies, such as acupuncture or homeopathy.

I should point out before proceeding that the truly holistic view, desired by most pet owners, involves looking at all options and choosing what works best with the fewest side effects. I'm a conventional doctor by training, and conventional therapies work well for many pets. Drugs such as corticosteroids and non-steroidal anti-inflammatory medications are not by nature harmful *when used correctly/holistically*. Some pets, especially cats, are more difficult to medicate then others; owners of these pets may choose to treat their arthritic pets "as needed" with long-acting injectable corticosteroids (although I avoid these potent drugs as often as possible). However, when you're trying to do the best, most natural and holistic thing for your pet, it's wise to consider all options before giving up and resigning yourself to chronic steroid or NSAID therapy for the arthritic pet.

Keep in mind that our ultimate goal when treating the pet with arthritis in a holistic fashion is to achieve *true healing*, rather than to simply make the pet feel better. This can be done only when using natural therapies.

I believe that what I do — offering both conventional and alternative therapies to owners — is the best of both worlds. By knowing the pros and cons of both types of medical care, the owner can work with me and pick the therapy that he or she is most comfortable with and that is most beneficial to the pet. This is a good place to point out that *holistic* doesn't necessarily mean "alternative." A truly holistic approach is an attempt to heal the entire pet and not simply cover up symptoms. A doctor using a truly holistic approach chooses what's best for the pet and attempts to give it relief while minimizing side effects. Conventional drug therapy can be a part of the holistic approach to treating arthritis *if* the goal is to help the pet become healthier and not to simply cover up symptoms while ignoring the pet's well-being.

The problems I have with the conventional therapy for arthritis, which involves the long-term administration of potent drugs — such as NSAIDs, corticosteroids, and painkillers (analgesics) like butorphanol, tramadol, gabapentin, and others — are numerous. First, many doctors fail to make a proper diagnosis. Maybe they don't want the owner to spend much money on a diagnosis of the pet's problems. Maybe these doctors just decide the pet has arthritis, which they figure is easy enough to treat with corticosteroids or other medications that relieve pain and inflammation, and they simply hope the pet doesn't experience any serious side effects.

However, these are not excuses for failing to diagnose and treat the pet correctly. While arthritis is the most common diagnosis in older lame pets, other more serious conditions can also cause lameness. These other causes include, but are not limited to, bone infections (bacterial or fungal), bone cysts, bone tumors, fractures, ligamentous injuries (cruciate injuries), and joint instability (hip dysplasia, shoulder dysplasia, elbow dysplasia, and osteochondritis). Every doctor can refer those cases he or she is uncomfortable handling.

It is troubling that so many pets I see have not received a proper diagnosis but have been treated for months or years with potentially harmful "antiarthritis" therapies. A good number of these pets have never had *any* diagnostic tests done. Yet often a simple radiograph, a test that any doctor is able to perform, will reveal the cause of the pet's lameness. There is simply no excuse for failing to obtain a proper diagnosis before beginning chronic treatment of a pet.

So the bottom line is: before doctors condemn a pet to chronic corticosteroid or NSAID therapy, even if that is what the owner desires, we need to get, at the very least, a proper diagnosis and make sure that our treatment choice is correct.

*I hold the holistic belief that each pet is
an individual and must be treated as such.*

CHAPTER ONE

UNDERSTANDING ARTHRITIS

ARTHRITIS, OR, MORE CORRECTLY, OSTEOARTHRITIS or degenerative joint disease, is a common condition in older pets. *Arthritis* technically means "inflammation of the joint." So when we talk about arthritis, we are talking about an inflammatory disease. Inflammation is characterized by swelling, stiffness, and pain. When we treat pets with arthritis, our therapy must be designed to counteract these effects of inflammation. It would also be advantageous if the therapy could slow down the progression of the arthritis or, if possible, actually help the damaged joint to heal.

Most conventional therapies do a great job of treating inflammation and pain but rarely help the joint to heal. And in many cases, these anti-inflammatory therapies actually cause *more* cartilage damage (and with it, more arthritis) over time. Many natural therapies, conversely, not only relieve pain and inflammation but actually supply nutrients to help the cartilage heal and slow down the destructive forces of nature that act to destroy the injured joint.

As I stated in the introduction, because lameness caused by osteo-arthritis is commonly found in older pets, and because many doctors are uncomfortable treating geriatric pets, older pets are often ignored and improperly treated. Many veterinarians, instead of performing diagnostic testing to determine the cause and severity of the problem, and instead of searching for the least harmful treatment options, just try to make such a pet comfortable for whatever time the pet has left. These pets are often treated with corticosteroids or nonsteroidal anti-inflammatory medications without the benefit of a proper diagnosis. While nothing is wrong with making pets comfortable, assuming that a geriatric pet with osteoarthritis is on its last legs is unreasonable. Many older pets can look forward to months or years of good-quality living when doctors treat them as they would younger pets. There's also no reason for doctors to reach for corticosteroids or other potentially harmful medications, such as nonsteroidal medications, if more natural, safer alternatives are available.

Many older pets can look forward to months or years of good-quality living when doctors treat them as they would younger pets.

While conventional therapy for osteoarthritis raises many concerns, perhaps the greatest is that many veterinarians prescribe without making a proper diagnosis. It may be that these doctors don't want owners to have to spend much money on diagnosing their pets' problems. Maybe the doctors simply assume that the pets have arthritis, which they figure is easy enough to treat with corticosteroids or other medications that relieve pain and inflammation, and they simply hope the pet doesn't experience serious side effects. These reasons, however, are poor excuses for failing to diagnose and treat the pet correctly. Arthritis is certainly the most common diagnosis in older lame pets, but other, more serious conditions can also cause lameness. Bone infections (bacterial or fungal), tumors, injuries, bone cysts, bone tumors, fractures, ligamentous injuries (cruciate injuries), and joint instability (hip dysplasia, shoulder dysplasia, elbow dysplasia, and osteochondritis) are among the more common causes. I discuss these in chapter 2.

> *No decision should be made concerning the long-term care of your dog or cat until you know exactly what's wrong.*

WHERE ARTHRITIS STRIKES

As mentioned earlier, *arthritis* technically means "inflammation of the joint." In both pets and people, it is an inflammatory disease characterized by swelling, stiffness, and pain.

Joints commonly affected with arthritis include the knee, shoulder, ankle, elbow, and, most commonly in dogs, the hips. The joints between the vertebrae of the backbone (spine) also commonly develop arthritis. In most dogs, arthritis of the spine does not cause pain or discomfort. The same joints affected by arthritis in dogs are also affected in cats, although cats often develop arthritis of the smaller joints of the feet as well.

Arthritis results from erosion of the articular cartilage lining the joints. The lack of nerves in the articular cartilage is an important factor in the progression of arthritis. A great amount of damage to the cartilage can occur before the surrounding joint tissues (joint capsule, bones, and ligaments) become inflamed and cause lameness. Because of this, considerable cartilage damage is often present by the time the animal actually feels any pain and shows signs of lameness. Annual screening of the hips and spine, the most common joints affected with osteoarthritis, will allow for early diagnosis and treatment — before irreversible cartilage damage occurs.

THE JOINT AND CARTILAGE: A CLOSER LOOK

The components of the joint include the bones of the joint, ligaments from surrounding muscles that cross the joint space and attach to the bones, and the joint capsule, which encloses the joint. The joint capsule contains a thick protective outer layer, and a thin inner layer called the synovial membrane. The synovial membrane contains blood vessels and nerves and produces a special fluid in the joint called synovial fluid.

The end of each bone is covered with cartilage called articular cartilage, which acts as a shock absorber to protect the bone. The articular cartilage lacks blood vessels and nerves and depends on the diffusion of nutrients from synovial fluid. This fluid lines the joint space, nourishing the cartilage, and it acts as a lubricant and shock absorber.

With enough degradation of the cartilage, underlying bone may become damaged and the animal may refuse to use the affected limb. That's when the dog or cat begins to limp and its owner often seeks medical care. Some pets can still be helped with nutritional therapies to heal the joint, but others may have arthritis too advanced to actually allow for healing. The earlier the pet is diagnosed, the greater the chance for healing to occur using complementary therapies.

In addition to this general pathway for damage to the joint and its components, there are also specific causes of arthritis. For example, dogs with hip dysplasia have abnormal hip joints, which leads to instability. As the instability progresses, the body attempts to stabilize the joint by forming new bone around it. While this may sound like a good idea, unfortunately this new bone does not stabilize the joint but instead causes pain and inflammation.

THE ARTICULAR CARTILAGE: A CLOSER LOOK

The articular cartilage has a unique structure that allows it to handle the stressful loads placed on it as the animal walks and plays. The articular cartilage is made of both cartilage cells (the medical term is *chondrocytes*) and the tissue, called matrix, that surrounds these cells. The major components of this cartilage matrix are a type of protein (called collagen), water, and proteoglycans. The proteoglycan molecule is made of a central core of protein with numerous side chains of glycosaminoglycans (GAGs). There are several different proteoglycan molecules in the joint cartilage, including chondroitin sulfate (the predominant GAG in cartilage) and keratan sulfate. Glucosamine, a popular treatment for osteoarthritis, is a precursor chemical necessary for glycosaminoglycan synthesis. As I discuss nutritional treatments for arthritis, it will be important to remember the terms *glycosaminoglycan*, *proteoglycan*, and *chondroitin sulfate*, as some of the treatments attempt to furnish more of these molecules to help the cartilage heal.

As the animal walks and plays, a large amount of stress is placed on all the components of the joint. Biomechanical and biochemical alterations in the joints occur. With years of wear and tear on the joints, the cartilage breaks down and arthritis can develop. As wear and tear continues, the cartilage is disrupted and joint instability results. Chondrocytes, the cells that make up cartilage, are not able to synthesize enough of the proteoglycans to permit the cartilage to heal. As the chondrocytes become degraded, inflammatory chemicals are released, causing inflammation and further damaging the cartilage. The inflammatory chemicals also disrupt the proteoglycans. With enough degradation of the cartilage, underlying bone may become damaged, and the animal may refuse to use the affected limb. At this point, owners often seek medical care. Some pets can still be helped with nutritional therapies to heal the joint, but others may have arthritis too advanced to actually allow for true healing. The earlier the pet is diagnosed, the greater the chance for healing to occur using natural therapies.

This new bone and accompanying inflammation in and around it is called arthritis. Dogs with arthritis of the spine most likely develop this new bone and the inflammation as a result of degeneration of the intervertebral disks, the cartilage shock absorbers located between the vertebrae. Regardless of the cause, with time the joint instability and resulting inflammation occur. As the arthritis progresses, clinical signs begin to appear.

> *The earlier the pet is diagnosed, the greater the chance for healing to occur using natural therapies.*

It is worthwhile to point out that some types of arthritis can be prevented. For example, hip dysplasia is a common cause of arthritis in older dogs and even cats. With this condition, the hips are unstable as a result of genetic factors, environmental factors, or both. Some puppies show signs of hip dysplasia before twelve months of age. These dogs have difficulty rising and their hind-quarters sway when they walk. When the owners manipulate the dogs' legs, this may cause the dogs pain. Pets can be screened for this condition very early in life, and while many owners are familiar with the screening of breeding dogs at two years of age, others are surprised that puppies (and kittens) can be screened early in life. We routinely screen puppies and kittens brought in for spaying and neutering. Surprisingly, 40 to 50 percent of puppies we screen for hip dysplasia actually have the condition. Remember, these are "normal" puppies with no clinical history. They walk and play normally.

Under anesthesia, the puppies are radiographed for signs of hip dysplasia. Also, we attempt to physically "pop" the hips out of joint to check them for instability, which can indicate dysplasia. (I know this sounds graphic, but after we pop the hips out of joint, they go right back in at the end of our evaluation and the pet never feels any aftereffects.) The reason for early screening is that, if signs of hip dysplasia are discovered as a result of our radiography or orthopedic manipulations, surgery to repair or replace the joint is available. When the owner chooses to have the problem corrected early, it is rare for arthritis of the hips to develop later in life. This, then, is one arthritic condition that can actually be prevented early in life, either through surgery or careful screening of the parents before breeding.

It is enough to remember that osteoarthritis forms after months to years of wear and tear on the joints. With therapy, we not only relieve the pain and inflammation that accompany arthritis but also help heal the cartilage by supplying it with glycosaminoglycans. The therapies most commonly prescribed by doctors are conventional medications, which I'll discuss shortly.

*The best therapy for pets with arthritis is designed
to relieve pain and inflammation and heal
the destroyed cartilage with minimal or no side effects.*

CHAPTER SUMMARY

- Before beginning any treatment for your pet, be sure to get a proper diagnosis.
- The most common cause of lameness in dogs is osteoarthritis.
- A painful condition, arthritis is medically called osteoarthritis or degenerative joint disease.
- Osteoarthritis is inflammation of a joint, and in dogs and cats it is found most commonly in the joints of the hips and spine.
- The sooner the problem is diagnosed, the greater the number of treatment options available, the less the pet will have to rely mainly on conventional medications for relief, and the more successful the therapy.

CHAPTER TWO

NOT ARTHRITIS
but SOMETHING ELSE

As I mentioned earlier, lameness in pets is often caused by osteoarthritis. The years of wear and tear on the joints lead to destruction of the articular (joint) cartilage and the resulting sign of lameness in the aging pet.

Other causes too, some even more serious than arthritis, lead to lameness. For this reason, let me stress again that a proper diagnosis should be obtained before embarking on chronic therapy for suspected arthritis. Administering nonsteroidal anti-inflammatory medications for seven to fourteen days to see if the pet improves is certainly not malpractice, and can be useful in healthy pets to determine if the pet experiences any relief from the cause of the lameness. But continuing to administer medication for a longer period without establishing the correct cause of the problem borders on negligence, if not outright malpractice. In the next chapter, I'll talk about what should happen during your veterinary visit to allow the doctor to accurately diagnose the cause of your pet's lameness. For now, I want to present other conditions that could cause your dog or cat to act lame, so that you can see the importance of a proper diagnosis (these conditions are also listed in the sidebar on pages 17–18).

The list that follows is not intended to substitute for a proper diagnosis. It is a tool for you to use to help your veterinarian determine exactly what is causing your dog's or cat's lameness, once arthritis has been ruled out, or once the treatment for arthritis has been determined not to be the complete solution to your pet's problem.

An unusual case of misdiagnosis presented itself when Angus, a seven-year-old neutered male Rottweiler, was referred to me for acupuncture for presumed hip dysplasia. I estimated Angus, at 149 pounds, to be approximately 30 to 40 pounds overweight. He had demonstrated difficulty moving around and lethargy, beginning two to three weeks before our visit. Within the previous week, according to his owner, Angus had "staggered as if he were drunk" when he stood up from a prone position.

One of two doctors who had already examined Angus had diagnosed hip dysplasia based on breed, age, physical examination, and a radiograph (X-ray). He had prescribed a nonsteroidal drug for Angus, but Angus's owner noticed no change in the dog after a two-week trial with the drug.

The medical history provided by the owner revealed recurrent staphylococcal pyoderma, a common bacterial skin infection in dogs, which was responsive to various antibiotics. His original veterinarian had mentioned the possibility of atopic dermatitis, a skin allergy, as a cause of Angus's constant itching and recurring skin infections, but had done no testing to determine whether the dog actually had the condition. Angus was fed a "premium obesity prevention diet" but did not lose weight while eating it.

The dog showed no sign of pain when I manipulated his limbs. Pelvic limb swaying, resembling a drunken stagger, was evident but no neurological deficits in either the front or rear limbs. Cranial nerve functioning was within normal limits, indicating no problems or diseases of the brain. He seemed to have mild but painless swelling of both front feet; fever was not detected. The dog had not been exposed to external parasites, according to the owner.

When I listened to Angus's chest, I noticed no abnormal heart or lung sounds; pulses were strong and regular. His abdomen and lymph nodes appeared to be normal, and his peripheral lymph nodes were not enlarged. Grade II periodontal disease was evident, based on the excessive tartar on his teeth.

His urine sample was normal. A review of Angus's pelvic radiographs, which the owner had brought in with him, showed that they were underexposed and offered only a frog leg–style view of the hip joints, because the films had been made without sedating the dog. The correct view — required to properly evaluate the hip joints — had not been obtained. Despite this shortcoming in his radiographs, it was apparent that hip dysplasia and secondary osteoarthritis were not the cause of Angus's clinical signs. As is typical with at least half the cases that come to me for complementary therapy for arthritis, the dog actually had perfectly normal hips that did not require treatment.

So what was causing Angus's problems? Based on his sudden onset of lethargy and a swaggering gait, I ordered a complete blood count and a biochemical blood profile. These tests revealed high cholesterol, anemia, and very low thyroid hormone levels. The diagnosis was easy to make: the dog suffered from a thyroid disease, hypothyroidism, which caused all his clinical signs and abnormal blood results.

Angus did not need nonsteroidal drugs or anything else to treat arthritis because he did not have arthritis. I prescribed thyroid supplements and a weight-loss diet instead. He experienced complete resolution of his clinical signs, and his blood values returned to normal. To date, he is doing very well: he is walking normally and is near his ideal weight. And because hypothyroidism can cause chronic skin infections, now that his thyroid disease is under control, Angus experiences fewer skin infections.

OLD AGE

As you read this book, you'll gain at least three important points. The first is, as I've noted, that your pet deserves a proper diagnosis before receiving chronic therapy for an apparent case of arthritis. The second is that, if your pet receives potentially harmful medications such as nonsteroidals or corticosteroids on a long-term basis, this should happen only after all other, safer treatments have failed — and then only with frequent, careful monitoring to allow early detection of side effects, including intestinal ulcers, kidney disease, and liver disease. The third and final important lesson of the book is this: *old age is not a disease!*

So many pets have owners (and, sadly, even doctors) who do not care for them properly because they are just "acting old." With rare exceptions, abnormal clinical signs in pets have little to do with aging and are instead symptoms of disease. A normal older pet does not vomit frequently, eat more (or less), drink more (or less), or show signs of forgetfulness or lameness. These are symptoms of conditions that require prompt diagnosis and proper treatment. So even though the older pet has a higher incidence of disease, including arthritis, don't ignore your pet's limp because he is old. To do so is a disservice to him and deprives him of all that geriatric medicine can do for him during his golden years.

With rare exceptions, abnormal clinical signs in pets have little to do with aging and are instead symptoms of disease.

Old age is not a disease. When any pet, regardless of age, acts differently than normal, please seek immediate professional care.

TRAUMA

Whether or not you've witnessed physical trauma to your dog or cat, your pet's lameness may be due to some simple injury. To ease your pet's pain and prevent complications, it is important that any lameness lasting more than a day or two be diagnosed and treated. Fractures, dislocations, and soft tissue injury typically result from trauma to your pet's musculoskeletal system.

Fractures and Dislocations

Fractures and dislocations are most often the result of trauma, although bone infections, nutritional diseases, and cancer can weaken the bone enough to cause fractures and resulting lameness. Trauma is usually readily recognized by the owner, making the diagnosis easy and unlikely to be confused with arthritis. However, some congenital disorders (described on pages 25–28) cause joint dislocations and result in lameness without trauma. A thorough orthopedic evaluation, including a radiograph, most often results in early diagnosis and successful treatment.

Soft Tissue Injuries

Trauma may also cause soft tissue injuries, which are not always as easily diagnosed as fractures and dislocations. Common soft tissue injuries include rupture of the cruciate ligaments of the knee joints and tearing of the collateral ligaments of the knee joints, similar to those seen in people. Cats too are prone to suffer traumatic injuries.

Diagnosis is made based on the patient's history. This usually includes a sudden onset of lameness following exercise, often an activity that involves sudden starts and stops or the twisting of the knee joints.

Radiographs are usually normal, although the rare pet with subtle and undiagnosed chronic ligament injuries will have secondary arthritis. Under anesthesia, pets with ligamentous tears will show increased joint laxity (looseness) when the affected joint is manipulated, compared to the normal joint on the opposite leg. Some cases require surgical or arthroscopic examination of the joint, or advanced radiographic procedures such as an MRI or CT scan, before a definitive diagnosis can be made.

Curative treatment involves surgery *when needed*. Often surgery is not needed, since ligamentous injuries can respond remarkably well to natural therapies. I have found that recovery is enhanced when surgery is combined with complementary therapies such as glucosamine, hyaluronic acid, glycosaminoglycans, nutritional supplements, and oral fatty acids. Herbs, acupuncture, laser therapy, and other therapies can aid in healing and offer pain relief.

I have had a high rate of success in treating patients' cruciate ligament injuries by means of aggressive supplementation with herbs, homotoxicology medications, and laser therapy. Most of these patients did not require surgery, saving the owners thousands of dollars and avoiding the rigors of postsurgical care for the pets.

Some soft tissue injuries are minor, such as bruises, muscle tears, or a thorn or piece of glass in the paw. Usually these heal with rest and time.

NEUROLOGICAL DISORDERS

Several neurological disorders cause dogs to show signs similar to those of arthritis.

Intervertebral Disk Disease

This disease causes varying degrees of paralysis, pain, or both, rather than true lameness. Still, since the pain from a protruding disk can lead to decreased mobility, it may cause a pet to move slowly and appear to be lame. Disk disease is most common in smaller breeds of dogs, such as dachshunds, and in cats.

> *Cases of disk disease frequently respond well to natural therapies, with less severe cases responding the best.*

Just like your backbone, your dog's backbone, or spine, is made up of bones called vertebrae. In between the vertebrae are shock-absorbing disks made of cartilage. These disks protect the ends of the vertebrae and absorb the impact, or shock, that is transmitted to the spine as the pet moves, runs, jumps, and walks.

Disk disease occurs when the disks degenerate. As degenerative changes arise, the disk becomes less elastic and calcifies; it can then no longer function as a shock absorber. With time, the center, and sometimes the outer part, of the disk degenerates to the point where it actually protrudes into the spinal canal, placing pressure on spinal nerves or even the spinal cord itself. This pressure causes pain, and in severe cases, paralysis, depending on where along the spinal canal the protruding disk is located and the amount of disk protruding into the canal.

Suspect disk disease if your pet shows signs of back pain or paralysis of the front or rear limbs. To identify disk disease, the doctor usually sedates the pet and radiographs the spine. Calcified disks, when they occur, are easily identified. However, in more than half of the cases I see, a special procedure such as a myelogram, CT scan, or MRI scan is needed to locate the disk protrusion.

Treatment varies, depending on the severity of the signs. Low doses of corticosteroids or nonsteroidal drugs can be used to provide immediate relief from pain and relieve nerve swelling; cage rest is essential to allow healing. Surgery is recommended in severe cases that result in paralysis and in cases of chronic pain and discomfort. Many cases of disk disease respond well to acupuncture, laser treatment, nutritional supplements, herbs, homeopathics, and homotoxicology medications. Even if you can't afford surgery, other natural therapies are often lifesaving for pets with disk disease, so don't give up. Regardless of the form of therapy chosen, the less severe cases respond the best.

Wobbler's Syndrome

This syndrome leads to abnormal swaying movements of the hind limbs called ataxia. The typical gait of pets with ataxia resembles that of someone walking when drunk; the pet displays a swaying, wobbly movement or unsteadiness when trying to walk.

The condition is seen most often in larger breeds of dogs, especially four- to eight-month-old Great Danes and four-year-old and older Doberman pinschers. The underlying cause is unknown, although genetics, joint defects, and excessive nutrition when the dog is young are all possibilities.

Dobermans and Great Danes that walk funny should be checked for Wobbler's syndrome. The syndrome involves one or more of the following problems: malformed vertebrae in the neck, protruding intervertebral disk in the neck, thickening of the ligaments surrounding the vertebrae in the neck, and instability of the vertebrae in the neck area.

Diagnosis is based on clinical signs and radiographs. Your veterinarian will probably need to perform special studies, such as a myelogram, CT scans, or MRI scans, to accurately pinpoint the lesion. Mild cases can improve with corticosteroids, acupuncture, and nutritional supplements. More severe cases may require surgical correction.

Cauda Equina Syndrome

The lower back, or lumbosacral joint, is a common site of disease in dogs, specifically in the larger breeds. Cauda equina syndrome refs to any lesion, usually an intervertebral disk, that compresses the nerves in this area of the spine.

Suspect cauda equina syndrome if your dog seems to be in pain when she moves, is reluctant to jump, exhibits pain when her lower back is manipulated or stroked, or shows hind limb stiffness or lameness. Neurological signs such as dragging one or both rear limbs, paralysis, and urinary or fecal incontinence can also occur.

The diagnosis is made under sedation by means of a radiograph and by special tests such as myelography, CT scans, or MRI scans when needed. Conventional treatment controls pain with steroids or nonsteroidal medications and with surgery in severe cases. Acupuncture and nutritional supplements can offer alternatives to conventional treatment.

CAUSES OF LAMENESS IN DOGS

Osteoarthritis
Old age
Trauma

- Fractures and dislocations
- Soft tissue injuries

Neurological disorders

- Intervertebral disk disease
- Wobbler's syndrome
- Cauda equina syndrome
- Fibrocartilage embolus

Autoimmune diseases

- Lupus

- Rheumatoid arthritis
- Drug reaction
- Vaccine reaction
- Dermatomyositis
- Polymyositis and polyarthritis
- Thyroid disease

Cancer

Congenital disorders

- Dysplasia
- Mucopolysaccharidosis

Infectious arthritis

- Lyme disease
- Hepatozoonosis
- Calicivirus (in cats)

Other Causes

- Overuse syndrome
- Osteochondrosis
- Panosteitis
- Spondylosis deformans
- Gout

Fibrocartilage Embolus

This rare, ill-defined, and difficult-to-diagnose disorder most commonly affects larger breeds of dogs. In fibrocartilage embolus, an acute onset of paralysis results, usually occurring after exercise or exertion. Although the exact cause is unknown, the condition is thought to occur because a microscopic piece of the fibrocartilaginous intervertebral disk somehow breaks away and travels as an embolus that then lodges in a blood vessel supplying the spinal cord. The paralysis usually affects only one side of the body, depending upon the location of the embolus.

Suspect fibrocartilage embolus if your dog goes lame suddenly, especially right after exercise. Because no easy, specific test is available for this condition, your veterinarian will make the diagnosis from the dog's medical history, and from negative findings for everything else on routine radiographs. There is no conventional treatment that is effective, and most dogs recover on their own, with supportive care if needed.

AUTOIMMUNE DISEASES

An autoimmune disease is one in which the dog's body turns on itself. Basically, the pet's immune system can no longer recognize its own normal tissues and instead treats its own tissues as if they are foreign invaders. The pet forms antibodies against its own cells, wreaking widespread destruction throughout the body. Lameness is a characteristic of several autoimmune diseases.

Lupus

This is the common name for a disease called systemic lupus erythematosus, which is among the most common in the category of autoimmune diseases. In pets and people with lupus, antibodies are formed against a variety of tissues, including joints, skin, muscles, kidneys, and bone marrow (causing anemia, low white blood cell counts, and low platelet counts). Because so many tissues can be affected by lupus, resulting in a variety of clinical signs, the disease is often called the "great imitator." Signs can be vague and intermittent, and may resemble those of many other conditions.

Because lupus resembles many other conditions and is very difficult to diagnose, it is easily overlooked as a cause of chronic lameness. And while lupus is not a common cause of lameness in dogs, lameness is the most common sign of lupus in dogs, being present in approximately 75 percent of affected animals. Once other common causes of lameness have been ruled out, consider lupus as a possible culprit. Diagnosis is based on clinical signs and often numerous laboratory tests, since no one specific "lupus test" exists.

> *An autoimmune disease is one in which
> the dog's body turns on itself.*

Conventional treatment involves high, immunosuppressive doses of corticosteroids or other chemotherapeutic drugs. Complementary care includes supportive care in the form of nutritional supplements.

Rheumatoid Arthritis

Another uncommon autoimmune cause of lameness, rheumatoid arthritis stimulates a dog's body to form antibodies against its own joints. This crippling disease causes typical signs of arthritis, including stiffness that is often pronounced in the morning, reluctance to exercise, pain when the joints are manipulated, and swelling of the involved joints. Rheumatoid arthritis causes more discomfort than does osteoarthritis. Pets with rheumatoid arthritis may be so severely affected that they cannot walk.

Suspect rheumatoid arthritis if you notice joint swelling, severe pain, and morning stiffness. Diagnosis is based on laboratory testing, including radiographs of the joint, a negative joint tap for bacteria and other infectious organisms, and a positive rheumatoid arthritis RF (which stands for "rheumatoid factor") blood test.

Rheumatoid arthritis is treated with analgesics (nonsteroidal medications for pain), corticosteroids, and other chemotherapeutic immunosuppressive medications. Nutritional supplements that are useful for the control of osteoarthritis may also be helpful if your dog develops rheumatoid arthritis. Acupuncture that stimulates immune-enhancing points can be tried as well.

Drug Reaction

Many doctors feel that drug-induced joint problems, while rare, are becoming more common in practice. The immune system can react to any drug, as the body usually considers drugs to be foreign substances. A hypersensitivity (allergic) reaction occurs when antibodies form chemical complexes with the administered drug; these drug-antibody complexes are then deposited in the joints. The drugs most commonly incriminated are antibiotics, especially sulfa drugs, erythromycin, penicillins, and cephalosporins.

The diagnosis is made when signs appear and worsen while the pet is taking the medication, and improvement is seen within two to seven days of stopping the medication. Supportive care is given as needed. Genetics may play a role in the development of a drug reaction. Doberman pinschers are predisposed to develop this problem when administered sulfa drugs.

*Since medications can cause acute lameness,
it is important to tell your veterinarian about all medicines,
including heartworm and flea prevention medicines,
that you give your pet.*

Vaccine Reaction

Immune disorders, including immune arthritis, are among the problems blamed on the ever-increasing use of vaccines. Vaccine-induced immune arthritis is occasionally seen following immunization, most often after distemper vaccination in puppies, calicivirus vaccination (or infection) in cats, and Lyme vaccination (or Lyme disease) in dogs.

The general feeling among veterinarians is that, in a very small number of pets, the distemper vaccine may be involved in some cases of immune arthritis, as distemper vaccine particles have been found in some of the affected joints.

Suspect vaccine-induced immune arthritis if your pet shows signs of lameness soon after receiving a vaccination. The problem usually resolves on its own and does not seem to recur with adult immunizations. Immune arthritis is just one of a variety of problems that the unnecessary immunization of pets can cause. The holistic approach to immunizations, which utilizes vaccine titers, helps decrease vaccine-related problems while still offering protection against infectious diseases.

Suspect vaccine-induced immune arthritis if your dog shows signs of lameness soon after receiving a vaccination.

Dermatomyositis

This condition, which affects mainly young collies and Shetland sheepdogs, is characterized by a skin condition and muscle inflammation. The cause is unknown, but dermatomyositis appears to be an autoimmune disease. Mildly affected dogs recover spontaneously, but more seriously affected pets may require treatment with immunosuppressive medications.

Polymyositis and Polyarthritis

Polymyositis is an autoimmune disease in which antibodies that attack the pet's muscle tissues are formed. Polyarthritis is a disease involving the formation of antibodies that attack the pet's joints. Both polymyositis and polyarthritis may occur in the same pet simultaneously.

Suspect polymyositis when you see stiffness and poor exercise tolerance. Muscle atrophy and pain may be present as well. Diagnosis is made by doing muscle biopsies, analyzing joint fluid, and ruling out other diseases. Conventional therapy is the same as for other immune-related disorders; complementary therapies can help regulate the immune system and relieve pain.

While rare, immune-mediated polyarthritis does occur in both dogs and cats. I have had excellent results in several of my patients afflicted with this condition by treating them with a combination of short-term conventional medications and lifelong supplementation with herbs, homeopathic and homotoxicologic medications, and nutritional supplements.

Thyroid Disease

Hypothyroidism, or low-thyroid disease, is probably the most common endocrine (hormonal) disease veterinarians diagnose in dogs. It is extremely rare in cats and, when it occurs, is usually a temporary complication following treatment for hyperthyroidism. Commonly considered an autoimmune disease, it causes the dog's body to form antibodies against its own thyroid glands. The presence of these antibodies prompts the thyroid gland to produce too little of the thyroid hormone.

Thyroid disease is underdiagnosed and is often the cause of a host of chronic diseases in dogs. When I was in school, we learned that the "classic signs" of hypothyroidism in dogs were obesity, hair loss, and the pet's tendency to seek warm places. Over the last few years, doctors have discovered that thyroid disease can have clinical signs like those of *any* number of diseases. Rarely do I see a pet with the "classic signs" of thyroid disease.

Angus, the Rottweiler I described at the beginning of this chapter, is an unusual example of hypothyroidism, and he demonstrates the idea that another disorder can cause signs that resemble those of arthritis. A dog's failure to respond to the appropriate dose of nonsteroidal medication should prompt a search for another disorder, as just about every dog with arthritis quickly improves with nonsteroidal medication. Because other disorders can cause arthritis-like symptoms, proper diagnostic testing is imperative, so that your veterinarian can make the correct diagnosis and offer the best treatment, as I discuss in the next chapter.

CANCER

Several cancers affect the bones of pets, and the resulting lameness can appear to signal arthritis. Most bone cancer tumors are primary tumors arising from the bone, rather than metastatic tumors that have spread from other locations in the body. Each year an estimated eight thousand to ten thousand dogs are diagnosed with bone cancer in the United States. Bone cancer does occur in cats but is very rare.

The most common tumors affecting bones, joints, and the surrounding soft tissues in dogs are osteosarcoma, chondrosarcoma, fibrosarcoma, and liposarcoma, as well as histiocytosis, which is found most often in Bernese mountain dogs. Osteosarcoma, however, is the most common tumor affecting the bones of dogs, accounting for 85 to 90 percent of all bone tumors, and it usually develops only in middle-aged dogs of the larger breeds. The bones most commonly diseased with osteosarcoma include the radius (forearm), humerus (upper arm), tibia (shin bone), and femur (upper leg bone).

If your pet has a swollen limb, immediately have it examined for bone cancer. Diagnosis is made by means of radiographs and a bone biopsy. If your veterinarian diagnoses bone cancer in your dog, insist on a chest radiograph to detect the spread of the tumor before you submit your pet to a surgical procedure that would be unnecessary if the cancer has spread at the time of diagnosis.

After early diagnosis, bone cancer, though not usually curable, is treatable with aggressive therapies. Conventional treatment requires surgical removal of the tumor, most commonly limb amputation, and chemotherapy. Some specialized facilities offer limb-sparing surgery in selected cases, which allows the dog to keep the limb after surgical removal of the tumor and affected bone. Complementary therapy includes a number of herbs and nutrients intended to stimulate the pet's immune system in an attempt to increase longevity and improve his quality of life.

I have seen dogs incorrectly diagnosed and treated for arthritis that, upon further evaluation, were discovered to have bone cancer. If your dog or cat does not respond to the proper therapy for arthritis within one to two weeks, the pet should be reevaluated and screened for bone cancer.

> *Complementary therapy includes a number of herbs and nutrients intended to stimulate the pet's immune system in an attempt to increase longevity and improve his quality of life.*

CONGENITAL DISORDERS

Present at birth, these disorders are usually considered inherited, although they may not actually show up until months or years after birth.

CONGENITAL ORTHOPEDIC PROBLEMS OF DOGS

The following is a catalogue of some of the orthopedic conditions diagnosed in dogs that may be confused with osteoarthritis. Congenital causes of lameness are very rare in cats; to date, I have never diagnosed a cat with a congenital cause of lameness. While any breed of dog could potentially be affected with any of these orthopedic conditions, I've listed the breeds most commonly affected. The conditions include hip dysplasia (which can occur in *any* breed of dog, including the smaller breeds, and in cats, but is most common in larger canine breeds, such as Labradors, golden retrievers, and German shepherds); shoulder dislocation (most common in smaller breeds, such as the Chihuahua, Yorkshire terrier, and miniature poodle); elbow dislocation (usually considered a large-dog problem); dislocations of the kneecap (smaller breeds are more commonly affected); atlantoaxial dislocation (a condition usually affecting smaller breeds, in which the articulation between the skull and spine dislocates); and dislocation of the temporomandibular joint of the skull.

These conditions can mimic arthritis. If not diagnosed properly when clinical signs are first apparent, osteoarthritis can develop with time due to chronic strain on the dislocating joint, causing additional problems. Most of these conditions respond well to early surgical correction when indicated.

Atlantoaxial dislocation: Chihuahua, Pekingese, Pomeranian, poodle, Yorkshire terrier

Cauda equina: German shepherd

Elbow dysplasia: basset hound, bullmastiff, French bulldog, German shepherd, Great Dane, Great Pyrenees, Irish wolfhound, Labrador retriever, Newfoundland, Weimaraner

Hip dysplasia: Mainly any large or giant breed, also cocker spaniel and Shetland sheepdog (sheltie)

Mucopolysaccharidosis VI: miniature pinscher
Osteoporosis: dachshund
Panosteitis: basset hound, German shepherd, and other
    breeds
Patellar (kneecap) dislocation: toy breeds
Shoulder dislocation: Chihuahua, griffon, Cavalier King
    Charles spaniel, miniature pinscher, miniature poodle,
    Pomeranian, wirehaired fox terrier
Wobbler's syndrome: basset hound, Doberman pinscher,
    English sheepdog, fox terrier, Great Dane, Irish setter,
    Rhodesian ridgeback, Saint Bernard

Purebred dogs should be screened early in life for the presence of congenital problems that can cause disease later in life. Dogs that carry a congenital disorder should not be bred. Several congenital disorders affecting the skeletal system can cause signs of lameness mimicking arthritis.

Purebred dogs should be screened early in life for the presence of congenital problems that can cause disease later in life.

Dysplasia

Hip dysplasia can occur in any breed of dog, including the smaller breeds, but is most common in larger breeds, such as Labrador and golden retrievers and German shepherds (it is rarely seen in cats). Shoulder dislocation is most common in smaller breeds, such as the Chihuahua, Yorkshire terrier, and miniature poodle. Elbow dislocations are also typically considered a large-dog problem. Dislocations of the kneecap more commonly affect smaller breeds. Atlantoaxial dislocation, which usually affects smaller breeds, is a condition in which the articulation between the skull and spine dislocates.

If not diagnosed properly when clinical signs are first seen, osteoarthritis can develop with time due to chronic strain on the dislocating joint, causing additional problems. Most of these conditions respond well to early surgical correction.

Mucopolysaccharidosis

A rare inherited disease in pets, mucopolysaccharidosis affects the joints' glycosaminoglycans, one of the building blocks of cartilage. Affected pets exhibit swollen, painful joints and often other signs, such as motor and visual deficits. Diagnosis involves special testing, and there is no treatment.

INFECTIOUS ARTHRITIS

Very rare in pets, infectious septic arthritis most commonly occurs as a complication of joint surgery or an open wound involving a joint. However, it can also be caused by infectious diseases such as Lyme disease, hepatozoonosis, and, in cats, calicivirus.

Lyme Disease

One cause of infectious arthritis in dogs, Lyme disease (also known as Lyme borreliosis), is becoming more common in certain areas of the country. Lyme disease is caused by a bacterium (specifically a spirochete) transmitted by the bite of a tick. The disease is not transmitted directly from pet to pet or between pets and their owners, as the organism must mature in the body of the tick and then be transmitted through the tick bite.

In people, a characteristic rash called erythema migrans is often located at the site of the tick bite. This rash is usually not detected in pets, because of the animal's fur. Lyme disease in people can cause disorders of the musculoskeletal system, nervous system, and even the heart. In dogs, the most common presentation is lameness. Many dogs develop a fever and swollen lymph nodes. Rarely do dogs show the neurological or cardiac problems seen in people with the disease.

The clinical signs resemble those typical of osteoarthritis, unless fever or joint swelling occurs. Pets living in areas of high tick concentrations are most at risk. To allow early diagnosis, have your pet tested for Lyme disease and the two other common tickborne diseases, ehrlichiosis and Rocky Mountain spotted fever, approximately thirty days after noticing a tick on the pet.

Diagnosis is achieved through clinical signs and a positive blood test. Dogs previously immunized against Lyme disease will test positive on the screening test commonly used for diagnosis; a second blood test can be used to find out whether that positive test resulted from the vaccination or a true incidence of the disease.

Because Lyme disease can affect both pets and their owners, tick prevention via tick control is extremely important. Immunization for Lyme disease is controversial among holistic veterinarians, and most doctors do not routinely recommend it for pets with limited tick exposure. I offer Lyme vaccine only to clients whose pets have a great deal of tick exposure, and to date I have noticed few acute side effects from the vaccine. A discussion with your doctor is in order if your pet has known tick exposure.

Treatment of Lyme disease is usually rewarding, and it involves the administration of appropriate antibiotics; acupuncture can be used to lessen joint pain.

Hepatozoonosis

Another infectious disease, hepatozoonosis, is also caused by a small parasitic organism, this one called a coccidian. While found throughout the world, the coccidian is most common along the U.S. Gulf Coast. Transmission occurs when the pet ingests the tick that carries the coccidian organism, unlike in most tick-related diseases, which result from the tick biting the pet.

Suspect hepatozoonosis if you have seen ticks on your pet in the past — or you live along or have recently visited the U.S. Gulf Coast — and you detect intermittent signs of the disease. Although the signs will vary in infected dogs, typical signs for hepatozoonosis include fever, weight loss, stiffness, discharge from the eyes and nose, and pain localized in the rear legs or spine. Signs appear periodically, and some dogs seem to recover for a period of time before symptoms return.

Diagnosis requires a high likelihood for the disease because the signs are vague and not specific to hepatozoonosis. For this reason, the disease is easily misdiagnosed. Radiographs can suggest the presence of this disease and can rule out simple osteoarthritis, although both conditions can exist together. Blood tests are also suggestive, but making a definitive diagnosis requires seeing the coccidial organism in biopsied tissue or in the blood.

No one medicine is perfect for treating hepatozoonosis, and in fact, the disease may be difficult if not impossible to cure. Treatment involves antibiotics and nonsteroidal medication for pain relief. Also consider complementary therapies to boost the immune system and relieve pain.

Calicivirus

Feline calicivirus is the cause of up to 50 percent of upper respiratory infections in cats. Its primary symptoms resemble those of a head cold in humans, such as fever, sneezing, and nasal discharge. Other symptoms can include runny eyes, ulceration of the mouth, and lameness, but some infected cats are asymptomatic. A small number of infected cats develop infectious arthritis, and those cats may not exhibit respiratory infection symptoms. Cats can become infected by direct contact with a carrier cat through discharge from the eyes, nose, or mouth, or indirectly through contaminated food bowls, bedding, and so on. Calicivirus is difficult to diagnose without specific tests because its symptoms are similar to those of other respiratory diseases. There is no specific treatment; supportive care with herbs and homeopathics — and antibiotics, if needed — can be helpful.

OTHER CAUSES

Overuse Syndrome

This condition is caused by an owner pushing the pet beyond its limits. More a problem in people and in very active dogs, overuse syndrome occurs in joints subject to repetitive strain — the hips, knees, ankles, and wrists. The more wear and tear on a joint, the more likely the joint will suffer inflammation and damage. Simply resting the joint allows healing. A short course of a nonsteroidal medication, acupuncture, or other complementary therapy can help as well.

The case of Missy comes to mind when I think of overuse syndrome. Missy is a middle-aged Shetland sheepdog (sheltie) with confirmed hip dysplasia and mild secondary osteoarthritis. She is doing well on nutritional supplements, including glucosamine, chondroitin, vitamin C, and omega-3 fatty acids.

The problem is not Missy so much as her owner, who loves to play hard with the dog. Her daily routine is to run Missy in the park for hours on end. The next day Missy is sore, reluctant to move, and often miserable. With two or three days of rest, however, she is back to normal.

While dogs with osteoarthritis can and should exercise (see chapter 8), Missy's owner obviously pushes her much too hard. When this happens, the dog pays the price later. By undertaking less strenuous exercise, and in this way minimizing the stress on Missy's hips, the owner could prevent Missy from suffering after her day at the park. By educating the owners of dogs with problems like Missy's, and by discovering what levels of exercise are best for these dogs, we can maximize their enjoyment as pets without causing them undue suffering.

Osteochondrosis

A common cause of lameness in large-breed puppies, this condition has been linked to rapid growth, overexertion, and excessive use of calcium supplements.

Osteochondrosis refers to a condition of unknown origin characterized by abnormal cartilage development in a young, growing dog. In pets with osteochondrosis, the growing cartilage fails to develop normally. Thickening of the joint cartilage occurs, and microscopic fissures and fractures subsequently develop. With normal stress on the abnormal cartilage as the puppy runs and plays, a tiny flap of cartilage can separate from the remaining joint cartilage covering the ends of the bones that make up the joint. The flap may calcify with time, which is easy to see when the joint is radiographed.

The exact reason why some puppies develop osteochondrosis is not known. Several theories have been proposed to explain the possible cause, including some relating to genetics, trauma, and nutrition. Trauma is mainly a disease of rapidly growing large-breed puppies that tend to be rambunctious (the owners of these breeds readily attest to their rambunctiousness!). An overabundance of nutrients may trigger the condition, as many of these puppies have been overfed to produce extremely rapid growth, and many have also received excessive calcium in their diets.

Vitamin C deficiency has been shown to cause osteochondrosis, although this is unlikely to occur in dogs because they, unlike people, manufacture their own vitamin C. Still many holistic doctors feel that giving additional vitamin C to growing puppies can prevent the occurrence of osteochondrosis and other problems, such as hip dysplasia; conventional veterinarians refute these claims.

Osteochondrosis *refers to a condition of unknown origin characterized by abnormal cartilage development in a young, growing dog.*

One holistic veterinarian recommends giving vitamin C to pregnant female dogs, and then to the newborn puppies, as a potential preventive measure. He also uses vitamin C in his patients with osteoarthritis and osteochondrosis in an effort to encourage healing of the cartilage. Since the exact amount of vitamin C needed is unknown, the doctor recommends slowly increasing the amount given until the level is reached at which mild diarrhea occurs (what is known as the bowel tolerance level), then reducing the dose slightly until the diarrhea disappears. This dose at which the diarrhea disappears becomes the therapeutic dose to use for that pet.

The joint most commonly affected with osteochondrosis is the shoulder joint. In many puppies, both joints are affected, even when the dog is lame in only one leg at the time of initial diagnosis. Other joints that may be affected include the elbow joint (often difficult to diagnose without special radiographic testing, such as an MRI), knee joint, and ankle joint. Radiographs of both the affected and the opposing, seemingly unaffected, joints are recommended. Often either special X-rays or surgical exploration of the joint is needed to allow proper diagnosis, especially in early cases, when joint problems do not show up on the radiographs.

Suspect osteochondrosis if your dog suffers acute lameness initiated by a recent mild traumatic event, such as catching a ball. The lameness may resolve on its own or with the use of nonsteroidal medication but will return soon after. Physical examination may prompt mild pain when the joint is manipulated. Due to the high incidence of osteochondrosis in rapidly growing larger-breed puppies, this condition remains uppermost on the list of possible diagnoses when a lame puppy is examined.

Treatment involves surgically removing the damaged cartilage and any joint flaps identified in the joint. Your dog will benefit greatly from the preoperative and postoperative use of nutritional supplements designed to aid in cartilage repair, pain relief, and inflammation relief, such as glucosamines, glycosaminoglycans, and chondroitin. Animals with osteochondrosis should not be bred, because the disease may be inherited.

Panosteitis

This condition causes lameness in the limbs of young large-breed dogs, especially the German shepherd, and is often difficult to diagnose in its earliest stages. Lameness typically lasts one to two months then resolves on its own, often to return in the same limb or another limb. The cause is unknown but suspected to be a result of genetics, metabolic diseases, blood vessel problems, or allergy.

In panosteitis, new bone grows in the marrow cavity of the bones of the limbs, causing pain, lameness, and sometimes fever. Radiographs may be normal if taken at the first signs of pain, but follow-up films taken a few weeks later usually reveal the problem.

The disease goes away after several months, but affected puppies are uncomfortable, and medications can be used to control pain. Nutritional supplements and acupuncture may also be helpful.

Spondylosis Deformans

Called ankylosing spondylitis in people, spondylosis deformans — or spondylosis for short — is an extremely common disorder in older dogs of any breed. In this condition, extra bone grows below the spine in response to chronic wear and tear, causing what is basically considered arthritis of the spine. But even when spondylosis is found, it may or may not cause lameness.

Suspect spondylosis if your older dog is stiff when getting up or lying down and does not want to jump. A diagnosis is easily made with spinal radiographs and by ruling out other causes of lameness. Most pets require no specific treatment, and certainly not drugs, unless they show clinical signs. For asymptomatic pets, I usually prescribe a nutritional supplement (such as glucosamine and chondroitin or hyaluronic acid) and omega-3 fatty acids to provide nourishment for the cartilage. Laser therapy, herbs, homotoxicology medications, and acupuncture can be used as needed to control pain.

Gout

Although somewhat common in people, gout is extremely rare in pets. It occurs when sodium urate crystals form in the joints, and a diagnosis is made by radiographing the joints and by aspirating them. The substance taken from the joints is examined microscopically to check for the crystals. Conventional therapy relies on antigout medication and changing the dog's diet to decrease urate crystal formation.

Miscellaneous Causes of Lameness

A number of rare peculiarities can manifest in a degree of lameness. For example, Doberman pinschers can be afflicted with a condition called dancing Doberman disease. Affected dogs hold up one rear limb while standing, often alternating with the opposite rear limb in a dancing motion. The cause is unknown but genetics is suspected; there is no treatment. This and other rare and peculiar problems are diagnosed only on the basis of known breed-specific problems after ruling out just about every other possibility.

Now that you've seen the number of conditions that can mimic osteoarthritis, and you understand why establishing a proper diagnosis early in the course of the disease is critical, let's talk, in the next chapter, about what to expect during your visit with your pet's doctor.

CHAPTER SUMMARY

- Osteoarthritis is the most common cause of lameness in dogs, but it's not the only cause.
- The true cause of your dog or cat's lameness must be diagnosed professionally.
- Old age is not a reason to ignore your pet's lameness.
- Consider other causes if your pet's signs do not match those of osteoarthritis.
- Look for other causes if your pet's signs do not go away after she takes arthritis medication for one week.
- Some, but not all, causes of lameness in dogs are breed specific.

CHAPTER THREE

WHAT CAN I EXPECT
at MY VETERINARY VISIT?

WHAT SHOULD YOU EXPECT when you visit your veterinarian with a pet showing signs of lameness?

Unfortunately, that depends on your doctor.

A doctor who is 100 percent conventional — whose mind is closed to complementary therapies — will have one approach, while a doctor who is 100 percent alternative, whose mind is closed to conventional therapies, will offer a totally different treatment plan. The conventional doctor won't be open to using therapies such as acupuncture, herbal medicine, and nutritional supplements. Instead, he or she will prefer to use unlimited medications and will often recommend surgery. This doctor may also offer little in the way of diagnostics, preferring instead to try various medications and take a "wait and see" approach.

Conversely, the doctor who practices only alternative medicine will probably not be open to using approved medications for short-term pain and inflammation relief, and may be totally opposed to any form of surgery. And a doctor like this one may use relatively little conventional diagnostic testing, instead preferring to treat your pet on the basis of clinical signs or alternative diagnostic techniques, such as reflex testing.

I believe the best doctors are those who are truly holistic, who offer both conventional and natural therapy options of the sort that I present in this book. By being open-minded yourself, willing to doing whatever is in your pet's best interest, you offer it the best care possible.

My encounter with Jet, an eight-year-old male Rottweiler, illustrates the importance of a good diagnosis. Jet was referred to me for acupuncture. He had exhibited lameness and the typical swaying gait of a larger-breed dog afflicted with hip dysplasia. His previous doctor had sedated him and taken radiographs (X-rays), which verified that Jet had hip dysplasia with secondary arthritis. My examination confirmed this diagnosis. Jet's owner, who did not want to use medications to control his signs if at all possible, contacted me about using acupuncture on the dog.

I prescribed a regimen of twice weekly acupuncture treatments, in addition to nutritional supplements containing glucosamine, chondroitin, and vitamin C. After several treatments, Jet was obviously not improving and was in fact worsening. He developed a low-grade fever and exhibited decreased appetite, increased joint stiffness, and swelling around the joints. Jet's failure to respond to treatment indicated a need to reassess our initial diagnosis. While his referring doctor and I both knew Jet had hip dysplasia compounded by osteoarthritis, his new clinical signs indicated that something else was going on too. I referred Jet's owner to a specialist, who performed further testing that indicated Jet had lupus. He responded well to medication to control the disease. Since his owner preferred not to travel to my office for ongoing acupuncture therapy, we continued with supplements for his osteoarthritis to decrease his lameness.

PRACTICING HOLISTIC MEDICINE

Several different terms attempt to explain the concept of natural pet care, including *holistic care*, *alternative therapies*, *complementary medicine*, and of course, *natural care*. What do all these terms mean, and how can you use them to determine which doctor should care for your pet?

Before I give you my definition of *holistic care*, let me quickly define these other terms often applied to nonconventional therapies.

Alternative therapy means any therapy that is an alternative to conventional medical treatment. This includes treatments such as homeopathy, acupuncture, herbal medicine, and nutritional medicine, to name a few common ones. "Complementary therapies" include those same therapies. The term *complementary therapy* is used interchangeably with *alternative therapy*, but it is not really correct to do so. *Alternative* implies "something other than," but the term *complementary therapy* implies that the chosen treatment "complements" the standard treatment and doesn't necessarily replace it. Since most holistic doctors are open-minded about using both complementary therapies and standard treatments, the preferred term *complementary therapy* means that a treatment such as acupuncture or homeopathy will be used in conjunction with, and complements, the traditional medical therapy that may be prescribed. *Natural care* refers to the practice of using treatments other than traditional drug therapies.

In my practice, I often use a conventional therapy for a pet when it is in that pet's best interest, but I also supplement my treatment with a few well-chosen complementary therapies.

Your goal as a pet owner is simple: to do what is in the best interest of your pet. If that includes conventional therapies, such as surgery and drug therapy, so be it. If your pet is better treated with a complementary therapy, such as herbal medicine, homeopathy,

39

or acupuncture, that's great too. And this is what holistic medicine is all about: simply keeping our minds open and doing what is in the best interests of our four-legged friends.

In order to be open to doing what is in the pet's best interest, doctor and pet owner alike must develop what I call a holistic mind-set. Recall that, as I mentioned in the introduction to this book, *holistic* care refers to a way of thinking. The holistic doctor and owner view the pet in its entirety, rather than just blindly focusing on a set of problems or signs and symptoms. The goal of holistic care is disease prevention. As a holistic doctor, I prefer to "treat the pet" rather than "treat a disease" (at best) or "treat signs and symptoms" (at worst).

> *The true holistic mind-set considers all options and then chooses those that are in the pet's best interest.*

How do you and your doctor go about developing a holistic mind-set, and why is this even important? When we change our thought processes and become more holistic, everyone, especially our pets, benefits. Doctors and owners with a holistic attitude refuse to focus only on the problem at hand and, instead, consider total wellness for the pet.

As I've spoken to pet owners and given interviews to promote this book, I've often been asked why more doctors don't practice holistic or natural medicine. I believe there are several reasons. First, we aren't trained to be holistic doctors. Until recently, few if any veterinary schools have offered wellness programs and courses on disease prevention. We are just now beginning to see a concentration on wellness and holistic care in medical schools, and I believe veterinary schools will eventually offer this too, although it will take some time.

Traditional pharmacology courses focus only on traditional

drug therapies and ignore natural treatments, such as herbal remedies. While it is vitally important to know about the many wonderful medications we can use to help our patients, a few lectures on natural treatments would help expose young doctors-to-be to these exciting therapies.

When I was in school, we concentrated on the diagnosis and treatment of diseases through recognition of signs and symptoms. While it is important to diagnose and treat diseases, it's more important to prevent as many of them as possible and to focus on *healing* the pet rather than *treating* a disease. Unfortunately, doctors are trained to be "disease diagnosers and treaters" rather than "patient healers."

Second, practicing holistic medicine takes time, and a lot of it. While many doctors find it useful to book four or more appointments per hour, and they maintain this schedule with the help of a well-trained, fully leveraged staff, the holistic practice on a typical day books one to two appointments per hour! It takes longer to develop a complete patient history and personalize a wellness "disease prevention" program for each patient.

Holistic care takes time and can't be rushed.

Third, a large number of doctors believe that anything other than conventional medicine is quackish. I get a lot of mail from doctors upset because I propose treatments that have not been subjected to double-blind studies. While I too hope for the day when rigorous trials are funded for more of our natural therapies, I must accept the clinical data we have now and do what I can to help my patients. I don't think I need to run expensive tests to show that, for example, the ten-thousand-year-old practice of acupuncture has merit. This is one therapy that has stood the test of time. The use of glucosamine products, while scoffed at when first suggested forty to forty-five years ago, is now accepted practice for treating osteoarthritis and is something I discuss in this book. Yes, there are charlatans out there, and some natural treatments have questionable value, but by and large there is considerable evidence of success for most of the established natural therapies.

FINDING A HOLISTIC VETERINARIAN

How, then, do you find a really good doctor who has a holistic philosophy? You may have to do some research. First, evaluate your pet's current veterinarian. Is he or she open to natural medicine? Many are, even if they don't offer specialized natural therapies themselves. Your current doctor can treat your pet's basic needs with a holistic approach, referring you to a doctor who performs natural therapies when those are needed.

Most doctors, even those who do not offer services like acupuncture and herbal medicine, now use nutritional supplements, such as glucosamine, chondroitin, and perna mussels (I discuss these in a later chapter), as part of their treatment of arthritic pets. This means your own doctor may be able to offer your arthritic pet some basic natural therapy. Hopefully, this trend of using supplements as part of the treatment of diseases will continue.

Or to find a good holistic doctor, you can ask friends for referrals. If you know someone who uses a holistic veterinarian, ask that person for a referral. Or try asking at the local health food store, pet store, or natural grocery store. These places get requests for referrals all the time. (Such stores have referred a number of clients to my own practice.) Or consult your phone book for veterinarians advertising holistic care. Stores often have directories with ads of holistic physicians and holistic veterinarians.

You might also consider contacting the American Holistic Veterinary Medical Association. You can reach this organization at 410-569-0795 or www.ahvma.org, and ask for referrals to doctors in your area.

If your doctor is not a holistic doctor, find one who is.

No method for locating a holistic doctor is foolproof, but these suggestions make a good starting point. Compile a list of as many names as possible, and then make an appointment to talk to each doctor on your list. Because your relationship with your pet's doctor is key to your pet's health, select a doctor you get along with. Make sure the doctor is open-minded about a variety of conventional and complementary therapies, and that he or she places your pet's health first.

ASK THE VETERINARIAN

Whether in person or on the telephone, interview the prospective holistic doctor who may end up treating your dog. After explaining that your dog is experiencing lameness and that you want to participate in a holistic treatment program, ask the veterinarian the following basic questions and listen carefully for appropriate answers.

Ask: How do you make a definitive diagnosis of osteoarthritis?
Ideal answer: Under heavy sedation or light anesthesia, with a full orthopedic examination and radiographs.
Ask: What are your feelings about using drugs to control pain?

Ideal answer: Short-term use of corticosteroids or nonsteroidal anti-inflammatory drugs is acceptable on an as-needed basis and varies from case to case. Chronic use of these medications is limited to the very rare pet that does not respond to any other therapy. Also, it is essential to do regular close monitoring of vital signs, plus laboratory testing, both of which should be done every two to three months to allow early detection of serious and potentially fatal side effects, such as liver disease, kidney disease, and diabetes.

Ask: What type of diet should my pet eat?

Ideal answer: A diet of the most natural prepared foods (devoid of potentially harmful by-products and chemicals) possible, or a homemade diet (cooked or raw), is recommended.

Ask: How do you treat chronic cases of osteoarthritis?

Ideal answer: Preferably, supplements, herbs, homeopathy, laser therapy, homotoxicology, acupuncture, and conventional medications, on a short-term, as-needed basis, are prescribed.

WHAT TO BRING WITH YOU

To get the most from your holistic veterinary visit, you must be an active participant. Begin your participation before your dog's appointment by doing the following:

- Verify when your pet's lameness began. Be prepared with an accurate estimate of how long your pet has been troubled. If the problem occurs only occasionally, keep notes about the circumstances when the lameness happens, such as after exercise or only in the morning.

- Provide all of your pet's medical records, or at least the names, addresses, and telephone numbers of all doctors your pet has visited. If you are visiting this doctor for a second opinion on a diagnosis, bring the results of any tests that have already been performed, and radiographs, if possible.
- Make notes of all treatments you have tried, both conventional and complementary, and any effect these treatments have had on your pet.
- Be sure to tell the doctor about any medications your pet is taking, including heartworm medications and over-the-counter flea and tick prevention. Always bring in any medicine containers, even if empty, so the doctor can assess the prescription. Many times I find that the wrong dosage or dosing interval was prescribed, and this may account for the pet's failure to improve.
- Know the ingredients and amounts of all the food your pet eats.
- As much as possible, track your pet's bowel and urinary output and any other signs of your pet's general health.

THE VETERINARY VISIT

Once you've found the perfect doctor for your pet and have arrived for your appointment, it's important to understand what should happen during your visit. If this is your first visit, expect to spend thirty to sixty minutes or more for the initial evaluation and diagnostic testing. The visit is divided into three parts: the medical history, examination, and laboratory evaluation.

The Medical History

The history you provide is vital to your veterinarian's proper assessment of your pet. It serves as a guide to the areas of the body he or she should pay particular attention to during the examination, and the laboratory tests needed to arrive at a proper diagnosis. It is not uncommon for clients to bring me pages of notes they have made at home, as well as notes and medical records from a previous doctor, to aid in my search for the correct diagnosis and treatment.

Your doctor will typically ask you the following about your pet:

1. What is your pet's diet?
2. Is your pet current on dental cleanings and preventive care — such as vaccinations when necessary and parasite control programs? The latter include heartworm medications if needed and treatment substitutes for chemical products to control fleas and ticks, unless chemicals are absolutely necessary.
3. Are you concerned about any signs in addition to the lameness? (The presence of other signs may point to a diagnosis other than osteoarthritis in the lame pet, or may indicate additional medical problems in your pet.)
4. Have you been to another doctor regarding the problem? If so:
   What was the diagnosis?
   How was the diagnosis made?
   What treatment was prescribed?
   Was the treatment effective?
5. Have you done any home treatments? If so:
   What treatments did you try?
   Did they help?

The Examination

After asking these and any other important questions, your doctor will begin the physical examination. I like to break the physical down into three parts: a general physical, an orthopedic examination, and a neurological examination.

The general physical allows the doctor to properly examine the pet from head to toe. During this part, I ignore the primary complaint of lameness so that I can detect other problems that may exist. Sometimes other problems are related to the lameness; sometimes they're not. By thoroughly checking the patient over, I offer truly holistic care. For example, I may discover that the pet also has a heart murmur, indicating heart disease, or a tumor that may be cancer. These problems can't be ignored and may actually take priority over the original problem.

The orthopedic examination allows the doctor to evaluate the musculoskeletal system and focus on the primary problem mentioned by the owner. During this part of the examination, I observe the pet at rest to determine general body condition, limb position, swelling of the limbs, and pain when the limbs are touched (palpated) or manipulated. During limb manipulations, I also listen and feel for crepitation, a grating sensation that may indicate arthritis. I check to see if any joints have abnormal movements, which could indicate ligament injury. Then I watch the pet get up from a down position, walk, turn, and lie back down, looking for signs of stiffness, pain, or reluctance to do any specific maneuver.

The final part of the examination, the neurological examination, relates particularly to the affected limb or limbs. The doctor will focus on questions such as: Is paralysis present? Are limb reflexes normal? Can the animal return a foot positioned in an unusual posture back to its normal position? Since more than half of the dogs I see for evaluation of hip dysplasia actually have neurological disease rather than dysplasia and secondary arthritis, this part of the examination, which many doctors bypass, is critical.

The Laboratory Evaluation

The laboratory evaluation is often crucial in determining the cause of your pet's lameness. It allows your veterinarian to distinguish

47

among subtle clues that he or she detected during the physical examination. Yet the laboratory evaluation is often the most neglected part of the overall evaluation. This is evident because of the number of first-time visitors to my practice who have been treated for arthritis by other doctors with potentially harmful medications, yet have never had so much as a simple radiograph or blood test to determine the correct diagnosis and treatment. Laboratory evaluations may include diagnostic imaging, bone scans, blood tests, thyroid testing, fluid analysis, and sometimes surgery.

DIAGNOSTIC IMAGING

Medical pictures of your pet often reveal the cause of its lameness. These tests are performed using machines, sometimes in the vet's office and sometimes in a separate laboratory. Common images are radiographs, MRI scans, CT scans, and myelograms.

> *Anesthesia may be required when radiographing pets because in some states it is against the law for medical personnel to be in the room when radiographs are being taken.*

The most basic diagnostic imaging test is the conventional radiograph. This two-dimensional picture, created using X-ray irradiation, allows the doctor to evaluate the dog's skeletal system. When this test is performed correctly, most pets do not need other imaging tests to properly diagnose the cause of their lameness.

Modern radiographic machines are very safe and are calibrated to deliver only the tiny amount of radiographic energy needed to produce high-quality pictures. Most often, two views are taken to allow the doctor to assess the affected area by means of a front-to-back view and a side-to-side view.

MRIs, CTs, AND MYELOGRAMS: A CLOSER LOOK

MRI (magnetic resonance imaging) scans make use of powerful magnets to detect magnetic fields in the body; a computer then analyzes these magnetic fields and turns them into a picture. This test is especially useful in looking at soft tissues, such as disks and ligaments, which are not revealed on conventional radiographs. CT (computed tomography) scans, formerly called CAT scans, use X-ray energy to produce more detailed pictures than those produced by regular radiographs. Myelograms involve injecting dye into the body, normally the spinal canal, and then using conventional radiographs to show the dye. This test is used for pets suspected of having disk disease or spinal tumors. Any blockage or deviation of the dye column indicates the presence of a spinal lesion, allowing the surgeon to pinpoint where to make an incision. The dye used in a myelogram can, on rare occasions, produce side effects, such as chemical meningitis or short-term seizures, as the pet awakens from anesthesia. While side effects are rare with today's safer dyes, you should discuss any concerns you have about this procedure with your pet's doctor.

Because even the best-trained pet will not lie still while his joints are placed in odd positions, most pets must be sedated to allow proper positioning and to minimize the need for multiple radiograph exposures. Anesthesia may be required when radiographing pets because in some states it is against the law for medical personnel to be in the room when radiographs are being taken. Modern sedatives are safe when used properly and the pet is monitored carefully. In my practice, the sedative is reversed at the completion of the radiographic procedure, and the pet is fully awake within minutes.

Occasionally, a conventional radiograph fails to reveal any abnormalities, and the doctor may order a more specialized test, such as an MRI, CT scan, myelogram, or bone scan. Again, the dog must be sedated to prevent movement during these tests.

BONE SCAN

While not used as commonly in pets as in people, a bone scan may be needed if other tests fail to detect the cause of a pet's lameness and the doctor suspects any lesions that may be present in the bones. In this procedure, which must be done under full anesthesia, a radioactive isotope is injected into the blood.

> *While not used as commonly in pets as in people, a bone scan may be needed if other tests fail to detect the cause of a pet's lameness.*

Then, a special scanning camera is used to detect accumulations of the isotope at various points in the body, such as any areas of bone that show inflammation, infection, or tumors. A computer assembles information provided by the camera and produces a picture for evaluation.

BLOOD TESTS

Your veterinarian may use a blood count and blood profile to help diagnose diseases that may be the cause of your dog's lameness. Blood tests provide information on the general health of the pet, the presence of another existing disease, and your dog's tolerance for medication. For example, a blood test may reveal diabetes. While diabetes does not typically cause lameness, early detection of this hormonal problem will extend your pet's life by allowing treatment to begin before clinical signs are present.

Blood tests also allow the doctor to determine whether prescribed medications should be altered. The blood profile is important if medications (especially corticosteroids or nonsteroidal anti-inflammatory medications) will be used for any length of time.

Since the nonsteroidal medications that many doctors typically prescribe for pets with osteoarthritis can cause intestinal ulcers, kidney disease, and liver disease, determining whether your pet has any of these problems is important. If problems are already present, the doctor may decide to lower the dose of the prescribed medication or even use a different medicine. And since nonsteroidal anti-inflammatory drugs can cause these problems, the very few pets that must use these products on a long-term basis need to have blood tests at least every two or three months to allow early detection of potentially fatal complications from medical therapy.

While diabetes does not typically cause lameness, early detection of this hormonal problem will extend your pet's life by allowing treatment to begin before clinical signs are present.

External parasites such as ticks may be a problem, depending on where you live. Ticks can carry diseases, including hepatozoonosis, ehrlichiosis, Rocky Mountain spotted fever, and Lyme disease (all of which can be transmitted to you). When indicated, your doctor may order additional blood tests to help determine whether a disease transmitted by a tick bite is the cause of your pet's lameness. As noted earlier, dogs previously vaccinated for Lyme disease usually have a positive serological screening test. An additional test is necessary to determine whether the positive result on the first test is due to vaccination or the actual disease.

I routinely test pets with known tick exposure one month following detection of a tick by the owner — even if the dog is not showing any clinical signs. Once again, early detection of these potentially fatal diseases allows us to treat the pet before any problems develop.

When the doctor suspects your pet's lameness has an immune cause, such as lupus or rheumatoid arthritis, he or she may order special blood tests (ANA test, LE test) for these illnesses as well.

THYROID TESTING

Hypothyroidism can cause neurological problems that can be misdiagnosed as lameness or arthritis in dogs. In cats, hyperthyroidism may cause clinical signs that can be confused with arthritis.

FLUID ANALYSIS

Another common test for diagnosing lameness in dogs is a synovial (joint) fluid analysis. Whenever joint swelling is noticed, the doctor may insert a tiny needle into the joint and aspirate a small amount of fluid for analysis. The fluid is examined for the presence of inflammatory cells, bacteria, fungi, tumor cells, or immune cells.

SURGERY

Occasionally, all laboratory tests fail to produce a diagnosis, and your veterinarian will recommend surgery. If you are on a limited budget and cannot afford to have every possible test done, surgery may be a more affordable option for you. Arthroscopy and arthrotomy are the two common types of surgery.

If you are on a limited budget and cannot afford to have every possible test done, surgery may be a more affordable option for you.

Surgery permits the doctor to examine the affected joint in an effort to diagnose and treat the problem. This is most often necessary in cases where ligaments of the joint are torn, as frequently occurs in cruciate ligament injury of the knee joint. In arthroscopy, the doctor inserts a tiny instrument called an arthroscope through a small incision and examines the joint. In arthrotomy, the doctor makes a conventional surgical incision to open the joint. When practical, arthroscopy is preferable because the incision is smaller, there are fewer side effects, and postoperative recovery time is decreased.

Once your doctor has verified the presence of osteoarthritis by means of your pet's medical history, a physical examination, and any necessary laboratory tests or surgery, he or she will review the various treatment options with you. The next chapter discusses the most commonly used conventional therapies, followed by a chapter presenting various complementary therapies your doctor may prescribe for your arthritic dog.

CHAPTER SUMMARY

- To receive holistic care for your pet, you must seek out and consult a holistic veterinarian.
- You and the holistic veterinarian will work together to create the best treatment for your pet.
- Before your appointment, observe your dog carefully so that you can describe all signs and symptoms.
- Bring your dog's complete medical history and records of any previous diagnosis to your appointment.
- In the office, the doctor will perform medical, orthopedic, and neurological examinations.
- The doctor will run a series of laboratory tests and perhaps do surgery in order to provide a proper diagnosis.

CHAPTER FOUR

CONVENTIONAL TREATMENTS *for* ARTHRITIS

I'VE BRIEFLY DISCUSSED some of the many conventional treatments for arthritis, which include corticosteroids, nonsteroidal anti-inflammatory drugs (NSAIDs), and surgery. Is one treatment preferred over the others? Is there a best treatment for arthritis? Before I discuss conventional treatments in this chapter and complementary therapies in the next, I'll share with you what I believe are the perfect criteria for choosing a treatment approach for the dog with osteoarthritis. The therapy

1. should be cost-effective;
2. should be easy for the owner to administer;
3. must be safe for the pet;
4. must have minimal or no short- or long-term side effects;
5. should help the joint heal itself and relieve inflammation and pain.

No matter what approach you ultimately chose, it should meet as many of these criteria as possible. As you will soon see, natural therapies fill most of these requirements, but conventional medications do not and are rarely suitable as long-term therapy for most arthritic pets.

HOW CONVENTIONAL THERAPIES WORK

As I discussed earlier, osteoarthritis is a painful condition of the joints. The pain that pets with arthritis feel results from damaged cell membranes releasing chemicals that cause inflammation. At a minimum, the treatment selected must relieve the inflammation and pain. For the long term, the treatment should encourage healing. Unfortunately, some of the conventional treatments for pets with arthritis do more to relieve the effects of the arthritis than to help the pet heal.

And some of our conventional treatments are actually harmful to the joint cartilage. For example, most of the corticosteroids or nonsteroidal anti-inflammatory medications that many doctors choose as long-term therapy for pets with arthritis *inhibit* healing of the cartilage, causing further destruction of the cartilage and joint components. So even though pets medicated in this way feel better for a while, their condition is made worse. Many pets taking corticosteroids for prolonged periods of time gain weight as a side effect of this class of medication, and may develop osteoporosis, and this excess weight and bone loss put further stress on already damaged joints.

Many pets taking corticosteroids for prolonged periods of time gain weight as a side effect of this class of medication, and this excess weight puts further stress on already damaged joints.

INFLAMMATION

Since most therapies for pets with arthritis are intended to relieve inflammation, it's important for owners to understand just what inflammation is and how these therapies help relieve this side effect. Then we can discuss the common conventional therapies currently used to treat pets with arthritis.

Inflammation is caused by damage to the tissues and cells of the affected body part. When a tissue is inflamed, it exhibits any or all of the following signs: redness, pain, tenderness, swelling, and loss of function.

Cell membranes contain chemicals called phospholipids. If the cell membrane is injured, as occurs in the arthritic pet, an enzyme acts on the phospholipids in the cell membrane to produce fatty acids, including arachidonic acid (an omega-6 fatty acid) and eicosapentaenoic acid (an omega-3 fatty acid). Further metabolism of the arachidonic acid and eicosapentaenoic acid by additional enzymes yields the production of chemicals called eicosanoids. The eicosanoids produced by metabolizing arachidonic acid (the omega-6 fatty acids) are pro-inflammatory and cause inflammation, suppress the immune system, and cause platelets to aggregate and clot. The eicosanoids produced by metabolism of eicosapentaenoic acid (the omega-3 fatty acids) are noninflammatory, not immunosuppressive, and help inhibit platelets from clotting.

Damaged cell membranes in pets with arthritis release chemicals, causing inflammation.

Various drugs work at different stages to help decrease the production of the chemical compounds that cause inflammation. For example, corticosteroids work at two places in this biochemical pathway: they help inhibit the enzyme responsible for metabolizing the membrane phospholipids into arachidonic and eicosapentaenoic acids, and they inhibit the enzyme responsible for breaking down arachidonic acid into pro-inflammatory compounds. Nonsteroidal anti-inflammatory medications, such as aspirin and ibuprofen, work at another step in the pathway (the COX pathway, discussed in "The COX-1 and COX-2 Enzymes" sidebar on page 70) that is responsible for metabolizing arachidonic acid into pro-inflammatory compounds.

Now that you have some understanding of what we must do to effectively relieve the pain and inflammation suffered by arthritic pets, let's take a look at the two most common classes of medications currently used to treat arthritis. While both classes have their place when properly used to treat arthritic dogs and cats, for long-term management we must make safer treatment choices. And, again, if these medications must be used, it is imperative that a proper diagnosis be made first. The case of Scooby drives this point home.

Scooby, an eight-year-old collie, is a classic case of the failure to diagnose a patient's disease and of the administration of an incorrect treatment. His owner brought Scooby to me for evaluation. The dog's previous doctor had, several months earlier, prescribed the new nonsteroidal anti-inflammatory medication carprofen, known by the brand-name Rimadyl, for Scooby's presumed arthritis. Rimadyl can be a wonderful drug when used correctly, but more than 50 percent of the pets I evaluate for suspected arthritis have conditions for which Rimadyl should never be prescribed.

This was the case with Scooby, as he, unfortunately, was not improving. His owner saw no change in Scooby's gait and felt it was still painful for the dog to get up from a seated position. I asked Scooby's owner what type of diagnostic testing had been done to confirm the idea that Scooby really had arthritis. Had any radiographs (X-rays) been taken or blood tests done by the previous veterinarian? According to the owner, there had been no tests. Based on his breed (large dog) and age (middle-aged to geriatric pet), Scooby's previous doctor had guessed that Scooby suffered from arthritis.

I suspected that Scooby was not in fact arthritic. Just about every dog with arthritis quickly responds to Rimadyl and similar medications, yet Scooby had not improved and had in fact worsened. I was also concerned about side effects from the drug and asked Scooby's owner if any regular blood testing had been done to check for ulcers or liver or kidney disease. Scooby's owner was surprised to hear there were side effects from the drug, having always been told how safe Rimadyl is when prescribed for arthritis.

My physical examination and the radiographs I took gave us the correct diagnosis. Scooby was not arthritic but instead suffered from a condition called degenerative myelopathy, a degeneration of his spinal nerves. Unfortunately, there is no cure for this progressive disorder, but we were able to stop the administration of Rimadyl and put Scooby on natural therapies that help some pets with his condition. The moral of Scooby's story is clear: get the proper diagnosis first, and then use the correct treatment. Treating without the benefit of a correct diagnosis saddles the owner with unnecessary expense and prolongs the problem for the pet. Simply doing a few tests would have produced the correct diagnosis for Scooby much earlier. Fortunately for him, his nonsteroidal treatment produced no ill side effects.

> *No type of treatment, conventional or complementary,*
> *should be administered on a long-term basis*
> *without a proper diagnosis.*

Corticosteroids, or *steroids* for short, are the first class of medications that comes to mind when a doctor thinks about treating the arthritic dog. Steroids are also among the most frequently used and abused drugs in veterinary, and probably human, medicine. It's just too easy for doctors to reach for the magic steroid shot to treat symptoms without truly diagnosing and treating the disease. As a result, pets are often incorrectly treated for months or years before someone says, "Enough. There must be a better way!"

Many of my holistic clients think corticosteroids are horrible drugs that must be avoided at all cost, but that's far from the truth. These marvelous drugs can be lifesaving when used correctly at the right dosage, for the proper length of time, and in a patient whose diagnosis suggests a disease that can be properly treated with corticosteroids. The problem is that these drugs are often used improperly. Because they can aggravate an existing case of osteoarthritis by inhibiting the synthesis of proteoglycans and collagen (the molecules that make up cartilage), there is rarely if ever a need for their long-term use to treat most arthritic patients.

What Steroids Do

Corticosteroids do a number of wonderful things. First, they are anti-inflammatory and analgesic (pain-relieving) medications. They decrease inflammation and swelling, alleviating the pain caused by inflammation, and relieve itching. (Their ability to relieve itching leads many doctors to overprescribe them for pets with allergic dermatitis.) They are also very helpful in the initial treatment of patients with severe shock and neurological disease (spinal cord and brain injuries) because they reduce inflammation.

CORTICOSTEROIDS: A CLOSER LOOK

So just what are corticosteroids? Why are so many people in the health care field eager to use these miracle drugs? Corticosteroids, or, more correctly, glucocorticoids, are hormones produced by the adrenal glands under the control of the pituitary gland. When the body needs to manufacture more of its own glucocorticoids, the pituitary gland produces a hormone called adrenocorticotrophic hormone (ACTH), which stimulates the adrenal gland to produce glucocorticoids. When the glucocorticoid level rises, the pituitary shuts off the ACTH signal; when the glucocorticoid level falls, the pituitary puts out more ACTH. This loop keeps the body's production of glucocorticoids in balance with the body's demand.

But when we give a pet corticosteroids as a treatment, the pituitary gland senses this and stops production of ACTH so that the adrenal glands won't make any more steroids. This effectively shuts down the body's normal production of a vitally important hormone. It won't hurt the pet if we use a low dose of steroid for a short period of time, such as seven to ten days. But if we use more potent steroids for a longer period of time, and then suddenly stop, the pet's body won't quickly adapt to the need for steroid production, and serious problems may result. This is one of the potentially serious side effects that occur when we treat pets with glucocorticoids.

Side Effects of Steroids

The negative side of these wonder drugs is that steroids can decrease the ability of wounds to heal and increase the chance of infection if used for too long or at a high dose. Pets that truly need long-term steroid therapy also need careful, frequent monitoring to allow for early detection of infection. Steroids may also contribute to further destruction of arthritic joints by decreasing collagen and proteoglycan synthesis, making them a poor choice for long-term therapy in most pets with arthritis. And corticosteroids are immunosuppressive. At a high enough dose, steroids suppress the body's immune system. While this can be useful in combating immune diseases, in which the body attacks itself, an animal with a suppressed immune system is prone to infection.

> *Pets that truly need long-term steroid therapy*
> *also need careful, frequent monitoring to allow*
> *for early detection of infection.*

Commonly seen short-term side effects of corticosteroids that you should be concerned about include an increase in appetite, an increase in water intake, and an increase in urine output. These side effects are commonly observed in most if not all dogs undergoing corticosteroid therapy. They can also occur in cats but are much less likely to do so, with one exception: corticosteroids occasionally cause diabetes in cats.

LONG-TERM SIDE EFFECTS
OF CORTICOSTEROID THERAPY IN DOGS

The long-term side effects, which act on nearly every organ of a dog's body, can do serious damage to your pet's quality of life. Steroid use also upsets laboratory tests, making artificial changes in liver enzymes, white blood cell values, and thyroid tests, which may cause the misdiagnosis of other problems, such as:

- Heart and cardiovascular system problems causing hypertension (high blood pressure) and sodium and water retention
- Changes in the skin causing acne, infection, excessive bruising, atrophy (degeneration or thinning) of the skin, and hair loss
- Hormonal problems, including infertility, growth failure, adrenal gland diseases, birth defects, and miscarriage
- Gastrointestinal upset such as ulcers, pancreatitis, and perforation
- Immune system suppression and decreased ability to resist infections
- Metabolic problems such as increased blood lipid levels, fatty liver disease, diabetes mellitus, Cushing's disease, Addison's disease, and obesity
- Musculoskeletal effects, including osteoporosis, muscle weakness, and possibly further cartilage destruction
- Nervous system issues of hyperactivity and lethargy
- Vision problems, including glaucoma and cataracts
- Respiratory failures such as blood clots in the lungs

The higher the dose and the longer the therapy, the worse the problem, but even pets taking the medications for a short time and at very low doses can show side effects. While the side effects of short-term use are not harmful, many owners find them upsetting. Therefore, when corticosteroids are used as part of the treatment of the arthritic dog, try to use the lowest dose possible for the shortest amount of time.

The long-term side effects of corticosteroid therapy are a totally different story (see the sidebar "Long-Term Side Effects of Corticosteroid Therapy in Dogs" on page 62). Because the numerous side effects of corticosteroid therapy are significant, I use it only when absolutely necessary.

To be fair, reports about whether corticosteroids actually destroy cartilage, worsening osteoarthritis, are conflicting. Since corticosteroids do decrease the abnormal formation of new bone and decrease the destructive enzymes that occur with arthritis, some studies report a positive benefit for their use. Other studies, especially those in which the corticosteroid was administered directly into the joint (called an intra-articular injection, and commonly used for people with osteoarthritis), showed microscopic evidence of cartilage damage even after a single intra-articular injection. Regardless of the potential damage to the joint, the number of other potential side effects suggests that in most pets natural therapies should be used for the long-term treatment of arthritis.

Keep in mind that, because corticosteroids are potent antiinflammatory and antipain medications, the decreased pain from the arthritis may encourage your dog to be more active. Normally, increased activity is good, but an arthritic pet's activity should be restricted and monitored. Increased activity, coupled with the cartilage destruction that may occur with corticosteroids, will add to the joint damage.

Again, my intention in relating all these facts to you is not to scare you into avoiding corticosteroids, but to educate you. If owners don't mind steroid therapy, steroids can be used safely and effectively to treat the few diseases for which they may be the best therapy. But as I've pointed out, doctors frequently reach for the steroids without arriving at a correct diagnosis, or without first pursuing other, safer, alternative therapies. When it comes to treating arthritis, high-dose corticosteroid therapy over the long term is not the best choice.

COMMONLY USED CORTICOSTEROIDS

SHORT ACTING
Duration: Lasts 8 to 12 hours

- Hydrocortisone

INTERMEDIATE ACTING
Duration: Lasts 12 to 36 hours

- Prednisone
- Prednisolone
- Methylprednisolone (Solu-Delta)
- Triamcinolone

LONG ACTING
Duration: Lasts longer than 36 hours

- Betamethasone
- Dexamethasone (Azium)

Note: The actual duration depends on a number of factors, including the specific formula. For example, the acetate and acetonide formulas are repositol, meaning they can act for weeks and last in the body for several months (very long acting). These preparations are overused in veterinary medicine and are the most harmful when used repeatedly.

Safe Use of Steroid Therapy

As noted earlier, pets on long-term corticosteroid therapy must be monitored for side effects closely and frequently — usually every two to three months by physical examination and blood and urine tests. Because of the side effects of corticosteroids, pets on long-term therapy do not, as a rule, live as long as they would have lived had they not been on these medications. It is distressing to see pets with osteoarthritis sentenced to a shortened life of corticosteroid therapy when no other therapies have been tried. It's true that some pets, in rare cases, do not respond to any other conventional therapy, or to a complementary therapy, and must take corticosteroids for life. And with appropriate dosing and monitoring, even these pets can have a decent quality of life. But I would choose chronic therapy with corticosteroids for the arthritic pet only when all other treatments had failed over the course of a year of trying safer therapies, and only if my other choice were euthanasia.

For pets with arthritis that require corticosteroids, or whose owners want to use them on a short-term basis, I usually can lower the dosage when owners agree to try nutritional supplements and other complementary therapies for them.

NONSTEROIDAL ANTI-INFLAMMATORY DRUGS

NSAIDs are the second group of medications commonly prescribed for people and pets with various painful and inflammatory conditions, including osteoarthritis. There are many different NSAIDs for people and pets (see the sidebar "Common Nonsteroidal Anti-inflammatory Medications" on page 67). Acetaminophen (Tylenol) is another pain reliever often prescribed for arthritis, but incorrectly, as it has no anti-inflammatory properties.

Since dogs and, especially, cats have shown greater toxicity (usually increased gastrointestinal side effects) with most of the NSAIDs that are intended for humans, *the utmost care must be used when giving them to pets*. In general, they are not usually prescribed for pets. Instead, specific NSAIDs developed for pets are prescribed by veterinarians to help pets with arthritis.

Side Effects of NSAIDs

Like corticosteroids, NSAIDs work by inhibiting the chemicals (types of prostaglandins) that cause pain and inflammation. These drugs also have the potential to produce a number of undesirable and potentially fatal side effects, such as gastrointestinal bleeding, ulcers, kidney disease, liver disease, immune disease, destruction of articular cartilage, neurologic signs, behavioral problems, and even death. We don't actually know the incidence of side effects in arthritic pets treated chronically (longer than one year) with NSAIDs. Because many of these medications are new, notably Rimadyl and EtoGesic, more studies are needed. One study, however, has produced an interesting statistic: four out of six dogs developed stomach ulcers after taking double the recommended dose of aspirin for thirty days. Unfortunately, little information is available on long-term side effects when dogs are given the recommended dose of aspirin.

COMMON NSAIDs

Acetaminophen (Tylenol)
Aspirin (Ascriptin, Bayer, others)
Carprofen (Novox, Rimadyl)*
Celecoxib (Celebrex)
Deracoxib (Deramaxx)*†
Diclofenac sodium (Arthrotec, Cataflam, Voltaren)
Diflunisal (Dolobid)
Etodolac (EtoGesic)*
Fenoprofen (Nalfon)
Firocoxib (Previcox)*
Flunixin meglumine (Banamine)

Flurbiprofen (Ansaid)
Ibuprofen (Advil, Motrin, Nuprin)
Indomethacin (Indocin)
Ketoprofen (Ketofen)
Meloxicam (Metacam)*
Naproxen (Aleve, Anaprox, Naprosyn, Naprelan)
Phenylbutazone (Butazolidin)
Piroxicam (Feldene)**
Salsalate (Salflex)
Sulindac (Clinoril)
Tepoxalin (Zubrin)*
Tolmetin (Tolectin)

* Approved for use in dogs and often used "off label" in cats under veterinary supervision (injectable meloxicam is approved for post-surgical pain in cats). Tepoxalin also inhibits the 5-LOX pathway.

** Often prescribed for pain control in dogs and cats with cancer. The use of piroxicam has, in rare cases, been associated with the resolution and cure of cancerous tumors.

† Deracoxib (Deramaxx) is also a sulfonamide and can be contraindicated for dogs sensitive to the side effects of this class of drugs – especially blood dyscrasias and adverse effects on the liver and joints.

Note: Most of these medications are unsafe to use in dogs or cats at any dosage. Also, acetaminophen has no anti-inflammatory properties but can relieve pain. It should be used only under close veterinary supervision, if at all, as it can be toxic in dogs. Acetaminophen is toxic and even fatal in cats and should never be used in this species.

(Adapted from Hobbs and Bucco, *The Natural Pharmacist: Everything You Need to Know about Arthritis*, 36–37.)

FDA WARNINGS ABOUT NSAIDs IN PETS

In veterinary medicine, approved veterinary NSAIDs are used to control the pain of osteoarthritis in dogs, and some are approved for the control of postoperative pain in dogs. Injectable meloxicam is approved for postoperative pain in cats.

However, there are risks and benefits with all commonly prescribed veterinary drugs, including NSAIDs. Veterinarians and pet owners should be aware of the following facts:

- Oral NSAIDs are approved for use in dogs only. Although not approved by the U.S. Food and Drug Administration (FDA) for use in cats, they are often used in cats as well.
- Before dogs or cats begin NSAID therapy, a complete history should be taken, and they should undergo a thorough physical examination.
- Appropriate blood and urine tests should be performed to establish baseline data prior to, and periodically during, administration of any NSAID.
- Veterinary NSAIDs may be associated with gastrointestinal problems in dogs. See the sidebar "Possible Side Effects in Dogs Treated with Nonsteroidal Medications" on page 81.
- Usage with other anti-inflammatory drugs, such as corticosteroids and other NSAIDs, should be avoided to minimize side effects. Combining an NSAID with a similar drug (a corticosteroid or another NSAID) greatly increases the pet's risk of developing serious side effects.
- Patients at greatest risk for kidney problems are those

that are dehydrated (especially older pets), are undergoing diuretic treatment, or have preexisting kidney, heart, and/or liver problems.

Risks associated with NSAIDs are detailed on the package inserts and client information sheets of the particular NSAID.

(Adapted from the FDA website at www.fda.gov/animalveterinary/safetyhealth/productsafetyinformation/ucm055434.htm.)

THE COX-1 AND COX-2 ENZYMES: A CLOSER LOOK

Like corticosteroids, NSAIDs work by inhibiting the chemicals (types of prostaglandins) that cause pain and inflammation. While they can be very useful in controlling pain and inflammation, they have side effects, some more dangerous than others. Before I discuss these side effects further, I want to give you a short biochemistry lesson to help you understand how they can occur.

Earlier in this chapter, I talked about nonsteroidal medications that affect something called the COX pathway. *COX* stands for "cyclooxygenase," another enzyme in the pathway that breaks down the arachidonic acids in the cell membranes of the cartilage cells into chemicals such as free radicals and various prostaglandins, which damage the articular cartilage.

Two COX enzymes have been discovered to date: COX-1 and COX-2. COX-1 is found in various tissues, including the stomach, intestines, and kidneys, and has an important role in maintaining health. When arachidonic acid is broken down by COX-1, good, anti-inflammatory prostaglandins are produced. These prostaglandins keep the kidneys functioning normally and help protect the stomach and intestinal tract against ulcers.

When arachidonic acid is broken down by COX-2, bad, pro-inflammatory prostaglandins are produced. These prostaglandins (and other chemicals) are harmful and contribute to the side effects seen in some patients taking NSAIDs, such as ulcers in the gastrointestinal tract and kidney disease. Drugs that selectively inhibit COX-2 but not COX-1 are most likely to result in fewer side effects and to be safer for patients. Right now the move is on to find such NSAIDs.

Unfortunately, NSAIDs marketed as COX-2-selective inhibitors have not turned out to be as safe as previously hoped. There are still reports of significant gastrointestinal side effects, particularly in people and rarely in pets, taking COX-2 inhibitors. Additionally, since some COX-2 inhibitors work extremely well at inhibiting COX-2 while sparing COX-1, an unexpected side effect (heart attack) has been reported (as a result of excess thromboxane A2 accumulation). Two COX-2-inhibiting medications manufactured for people, Vioxx and Celebrex, have been removed from the market.

All NSAIDs, even those marketed as COX-2-selective inhibitors, should be considered potent medications with the potential to cause significant side effects.

In addition to the COX pathway, there is also the 5-LOX (lipoxygenase) pathway (and likely others we have not yet discovered), which is responsible for the production of inflammatory chemicals called leukotrienes. The biochemistry of inflammation and pain can be overwhelming, but the basic take-home point is that many drugs, such as NSAIDs (and homeopathics and various herbs, such as boswellia and curcumin) work by inhibiting the COX or LOX pathways.

Current NSAIDs available for veterinary patients inhibit both COX-1 and COX-2 to various degrees. Indomethacin and piroxicam have high COX-2/COX-1 ratios and result in high incidences of gastrointestinal problems (bleeding and ulcers). Naproxen (Aleve), ibuprofen (Advil or Motrin), carprofen (Rimadyl), meloxicam (Metacam), Tepoxalin (Zubrin), and etodolac (EtoGesic) have lower COX-2/COX-1 ratios, and as a result, are supposed to produce fewer incidences of gastrointestinal problems. While this may be true in some pets, COX-2-inhibiting NSAIDs have still been shown to cause side effects, including gastrointestinal disease, in pets and people. Tepoxalin (Zubrin) also inhibits lipoxygenase (LOX) and may offer better control of inflammation and pain, although this is hard to judge clinically in most pets. Aspirin has a higher ratio but produces an intermediate incidence of gastrointestinal problems, indicating that other mechanisms are involved in causing some of the side effects we may see in patients taking NSAIDs.

Nonsteroidal medications that are selective for COX-2 may be safer than other nonsteroidal medications but are not totally safe or without side effects.

Gastrointestinal bleeding can lead not only to ulcers of the stomach and intestine but also possibly to perforation of the stomach or intestines, as a result of prostaglandin inhibition. While it's good that nonsteroidal medications inhibit the prostaglandins (COX-2) that cause joint inflammation and pain, they also — as I point out in the short biochemistry lesson in the sidebar "The COX-1 and COX-2 Enzymes" on page 70 — inhibit the protective prostaglandins (COX-1) necessary to help prevent ulcers of the gastrointestinal tract.

These protective prostaglandins are needed to maintain the alkaline mucus barrier of the stomach, which prevents stomach acids from destroying the stomach lining. Inhibition of these protective prostaglandins decreases the protective mucus layer, making bleeding and ulceration more likely to occur. That is to say, while the nonsteroidal drugs are useful in treating arthritis, the same mechanism that relieves the inflammation and pain can also cause serious side effects in the stomach and intestines.

Side effects of nonsteroidal medications may include gastrointestinal ulcers, kidney disease, liver disease, and destruction of articular cartilage.

What is the incidence of side effects in arthritic pets treated chronically (greater than one year) with nonsteroidal medications? We really don't know; more studies are needed, as some of these medications have only recently become available, and I am not aware of any studies showing the incidence of side effects in pets treated with NSAID therapy for greater than one year.

According to package inserts included with NSAIDs, "Serious adverse reactions associated with this drug class can occur without warning and in rare situations result in death. Owners should be advised to discontinue therapy and contact their veterinarians immediately if signs of intolerance are observed." For information about specific veterinary NSAIDs, this link to the U.S. Food and Drug Administration website may prove helpful: www.fda.gov/animalveterinary/products/approvedanimal drugproducts/druglabels/ucm050105.htm.

The following information comes from the package insert that accompanied Celebrex, a nonsteroidal medication made by Pfizer and Searle for people, and which, as I noted, has been withdrawn from the market. (Keep in mind that Celebrex was supposed to be a safer NSAID, targeting mainly the COX-2 enzyme.) "Serious GI toxicity such as bleeding, ulceration, and perforation of the stomach, small intestine or large intestine, can occur at any time, with or without warning symptoms, in patients treated with NSAIDs. Only 20 percent of patients who develop serious upper GI adverse events on NSAID therapy are symptomatic. Upper GI ulcers…appear to occur in approximately 1 percent of patients treated for 3–6 months, and in about 2–4 percent of patients treated for one year."

The insert does go on to state that, in short-term studies on patients taking Celebrex for three to six months, only 0.04 percent experienced significant upper gastrointestinal bleeding, although the significance of this finding is unknown. While it appears that this product was possibly safer than other NSAIDs (which inhibit both COX-1 and COX-2), pay attention to the general warning signs listed in the insert regarding NSAID administration in general.

Only 20 percent of people who developed a serious gastrointestinal side effect *showed signs*; the other 80 percent had serious side effects but *did not show signs!* Unfortunately, we don't have good studies of our pets' responses to NSAIDs that we can compare to this study, but I assume that the incidence of asymptomatic pet patients is similar to that of human patients.

Let's look at some of the information put out by Pfizer,

manufacturer of not only Celebrex but also the popular NSAID Rimadyl, commonly prescribed for dogs. This information is excerpted from the *Pfizer Animal Health Technical Bulletin*, "First-Year Clinical Experience with Rimadyl (carprofen): Assessment of Product Safety, May 1998" and "Update: Two Years (1997–1998) Clinical Experience with Rimadyl (carprofen) August, 1999."

KEY POINTS

1. More than 2.5 million dogs were treated with Rimadyl.
2. The reported rate of adverse reactions was low, approximately 0.2 percent, in 1997, and 0.18 percent in the two-year study.
3. Approximately 70 percent of possible adverse drug events have been in older dogs.
4. Patient evaluation, including physical examination and appropriate diagnostics, is prudent before prescribing any medications.
5. When any medication is prescribed, owners should be informed of potential drug-related side effects and signs of drug intolerance.

Let's look at the last three key points, which I believe are the most important.

Key point 3 reports that most reactions to Rimadyl occur in older dogs. This is not surprising for several reasons (some of which I'll discuss along with the possible side effects of Rimadyl). First, most dogs with osteoarthritis are older dogs. Second, older pets are more likely to have adverse drug reactions because they have a decreased ability to metabolize and excrete drugs from their bodies, and because many older patients take multiple medications, which can interact with each other. Third, many older pets have additional medical problems, such as kidney or liver disease, which may be undiagnosed at the time a medicine is prescribed.

> *Older pets are more likely to have adverse drug reactions for two reasons: they have a decreased ability to metabolize and excrete drugs from their bodies, and many older patients are taking multiple medications, which can interact with each other.*

Key point 4 observes that every patient receiving any medication should have a proper physical examination and diagnostic testing (for nonsteroidal medications such as Rimadyl, blood and urine tests will usually suffice). Unfortunately, pets rarely receive the necessary diagnostics before chronic administration of Rimadyl is prescribed. If this drug is going to be administered to your pet for more than short-term treatment (three to seven days maximum), it is imperative that your pet receive diagnostic testing to uncover anything wrong that may increase its risk of adverse drug reactions.

Key point 5 states that owners should be told about possible side effects so they can recognize the earliest signs of any side effects, stop the medication, and notify the doctor. However, when it comes to Rimadyl, no owner has yet told me that his or her previous doctor discussed testing or side effects. Most owners are astonished to hear there are any side effects at all! This is no doubt due to Pfizer's multi-million-dollar advertising campaign promoting Rimadyl, which suggests that long-term treatment is now available to help restore your old pet back to its younger, more mobile self. In fairness to Pfizer, the ad briefly mentions that side effects can occur in pets taking NSAIDs. But based on my experience, owners overlook this caution, and their doctors neglect to point it out.

I would add a key point 6 to this list, stating that any pet that receives Rimadyl for long-term therapy should have ongoing examinations and diagnostics to allow early detection of any possible side effects. I require regular testing of pets receiving any medication on a long-term basis, before the owner can refill the prescription. To do anything else is bad medicine and potential malpractice.

The following is Pfizer's recommendation for the use of Rimadyl in geriatric dogs (six years of age and older). This too is excerpted from the *Pfizer Animal Health Technical Bulletin*, "First-Year Clinical Experience with Rimadyl (carprofen): Assessment of Product Safety, May 1998."

- Complete history and physical examination are necessary before prescribing Rimadyl.
- Definitive diagnosis should be determined so therapeutic response can be monitored.
- Baseline and repeat laboratory testing should be considered and are valuable in the geriatric dog.
- Follow-up communication between doctor and pet owner is important.
- Owners should be informed of clinical signs of drug intolerance (lack of appetite, vomiting, jaundice, and behavioral changes).
- Repeat laboratory values should be considered before refilling prescriptions.
- Recheck evaluations should be done after 2–4 weeks of treatment and then 3–6 months later if chronic treatment is needed.

I'm not picking on Rimadyl, because the information discussing Rimadyl could apply to any NSAID.

Now I'd like to discuss in further detail some of the side effects that may accompany any nonsteroidal medication prescribed for your dog or cat. I've already mentioned gastrointestinal problems like gastrointestinal bleeding and ulceration. Other potential side effects include kidney disease (also due to prostaglandin inhibition), liver disease (in mild cases, the pet displays elevated liver enzymes, and in more serious cases, the pet can show liver failure), immune diseases (anemia, low platelet count, skin diseases), neurologic signs (seizures, paralysis, unsteadiness), behavioral problems (hyperactivity, aggression, depression, sedation), drug interaction, cartilage damage, and even death. I'll discuss some of these in more detail.

KIDNEY DISEASE. Kidney dysfunction may occur due to prostaglandin inhibition as a result of NSAID administration. Dogs and cats with underlying kidney disease, usually older pets, are at greater risk. Any time a pet is dehydrated, the risk of kidney disease increases. Pets taking certain other medications, such as ACE inhibitors (enalapril, benazepril) or diuretics (furosemide), also have an increased risk of kidney damage. Pretreatment blood and urine testing can detect some but not all kidney problems.

LIVER DISEASE. The most serious side effect seen in dogs taking Rimadyl is liver disease. Two subsets of dogs with liver disease have been observed. In the first subset are dogs with elevated liver enzymes detected on a blood test. Most of these dogs are normal, and elevated enzymes were detected only during routine monitoring. The second and more disturbing subset is composed of dogs with signs of liver disease or liver failure. These dogs require intensive hospitalization, and death may result from this disease. One-third of all dogs in this class are Labrador retrievers. This may represent a true breed predisposition, or it may simply reflect the fact that Labrador retrievers are popular dogs and many of them have arthritis.

Rimadyl is the NSAID initially discovered to cause injury to the liver, but any NSAID can exhibit this side effect. However, since Rimadyl is the only NSAID I know of that causes problems specifically in Labrador retrievers, I prefer to use other NSAIDs in any retriever.

IMMUNE DISEASES. Anemia, low platelet counts, and skin reactions have been observed in dogs undergoing NSAID treatment.

NEUROLOGIC SIGNS. Seizures, paralysis, and unsteadiness have been seen in a small number of dogs taking NSAIDs.

BEHAVIORAL PROBLEMS. Aggression, depression, hyperactivity, and other behavioral problems can occur in pets taking Rimadyl or some other NSAIDs.

DRUG INTERACTIONS. NSAIDs can interact with other medications. These interactions can result in increased or decreased concentrations of the medications in the pet's blood, which may result in clinical signs of disease. Drug interaction is most likely to occur in pets taking medication for epilepsy (phenobarbital) or for heart failure (furosemide [Lasix], digoxin, or enalapril [Enacard] or other ACE inhibitors).

CARTILAGE DAMAGE. Finally, and perhaps most important, many of the NSAIDs destroy cartilage. They do this by inhibiting the enzymes necessary for the multiplication of the chondrocytes and the synthesis of proteoglycans. The newer COX-2 inhibitors appear to cause less cartilage destruction than other NSAIDs; time will tell if this holds true. Some studies reveal no cartilage damage in vitro (in the test tube) depending on the dose administered (some studies suggest that a low dosage actually increases the glycosaminoglycans, indicating cartilage healing). The significance of the in vitro tests has yet to be determined.

I've used Rimadyl as my NSAID example in this discussion because it was the first one developed and remains the one most commonly prescribed for dogs. However, even though other newer NSAIDs favor inhibition of primarily the COX-2 enzyme, they too can cause any of these same side effects.

To date I have not seen or heard of any breed-specific liver problems in pets taking EtoGesic or other COX-2 NSAIDs, which may indicate that these medications are better choices for Labrador retrievers with arthritis.

These products have been reported as safe for dogs for up to twelve months of continuous use, yet a number of dogs have taken NSAIDs for many years. We don't know whether more side effects will appear in pets taking NSAIDs for longer than the twelve-month period tested. Also, be aware that the safety margin in these products is narrow. For example, quoting from the EtoGesic package insert: "Elevated dose levels of EtoGesic at 2.7 times the maximum daily dose causes gastrointestinal ulceration, vomiting, and fecal blood and weight loss." Yet EtoGesic is supposed to be a "safe" NSAID.

Ideally, the first prescribed dose of an NSAID should start at the low end of the dosage range to minimize side effects. It is important to carefully follow the prescribed dosages if your pet must take NSAIDs for even a short time.

NSAID Use in Cats

While NSAIDs are approved only for use in dogs, to be given orally, most veterinarians use these drugs in cats too. It is perfectly legal to do this, as many conventional therapies for treating various disorders in dogs and cats are technically off label. The main thing to remember about NSAID usage in cats is that cats are much more susceptible to toxicity from medications, including from NSAIDs. As a result, cats should be given lower dosages in more frequent dosing intervals to minimize side effects and maximize safety. And as is true in treating dogs with arthritis, the liberal use of natural therapies is preferable. NSAIDs should be used only when necessary to control pain.

POSSIBLE SIDE EFFECTS IN DOGS TREATED WITH NONSTEROIDAL MEDICATIONS

- Gastrointestinal problems: stomach or intestinal bleeding, ulceration, perforation, pancreatitis, liver, and kidney toxicity
- Kidney disease
- Liver disease: elevated liver enzymes, liver disease or failure
- Immune diseases: anemia, low platelet counts, and skin reactions
- Neurologic signs: seizures, paralysis, unsteadiness
- Behavioral problems: aggression, depression, hyperactivity, and other behavioral problems
- Drug Interactions: phenobarbital, furosemide (Lasix), digoxin, and enalapril (Enacard) and other ACE inhibitors.
- Cartilage damage

There Is Good News Too!

While it may be tempting to swear off using NSAIDs, that is not my goal in presenting this information to you. Despite these potential side effects, nonsteroidal medications can be used safely and effectively under a doctor's supervision, most often for short-term pain management. I tend to use them for *temporary* relief (at about 25 to 50 percent of the recommended dosage — that is, the dosage shown on the label) while waiting to see results from natural therapies. This holistic approach combines conventional and natural therapies safely, to the benefit of the pet, while minimizing side effects.

Here is some of the good news about NSAID therapy:

First, the incidence of side effects is extremely low for pets taking NSAIDs, approximately 0.18 percent. I have not seen any side effects at all while using these products in my practice. However, I carefully screen my patients and use the medications only on a short-term, as-needed, basis.

> *NSAIDs are best used at the lowest dose*
> *needed to maintain patient comfort,*
> *and only on an as-needed basis.*

Second, compared to aspirin and other NSAIDs, the newer COX-2- and LOX-inhibiting medications have fewer side effects. For example, only minor gastrointestinal erosions were seen in dogs taking commonly prescribed, approved NSAIDs, but all dogs receiving aspirin had gastrointestinal hemorrhages. These approved medications are preferable to aspirin therapy for the arthritic dog.

NSAIDs are best used at the lowest dose needed to maintain patient comfort, and only on an as-needed basis.

Safe Use of NSAIDs

As I've noted, NSAIDs can be used safely and effectively for short-term pain management — for five to seven days. This is true for pets not on any other medications, and for pets without other diseases, after the doctor has taken a careful history, examined the pet, and done laboratory tests.

I prescribe NSAIDs at a reduced dose when the pet is having a particularly painful day. My general protocol is to rely on supplements, herbs, homotoxicologics, and laser therapy, using NSAIDs only on bad days and, if possible, at about one-quarter to one-half the label dosage.

For long-term use, I prescribe NSAIDs as a primary therapy only if *all other treatments have failed and the owner has been warned about potential side effects*. In such instances, I monitor patients frequently (every two to three months) for side effects (monitoring includes physical examinations and blood and urine tests). In some cases, I prescribe protective medications to decrease gastrointestinal side effects, which I'll say more about in a moment. In effect, we try to make the patient comfortable and help him have a good quality of life, at the risk of causing side effects and even death in that pet.

The best advice I can offer about using nonsteroidal medications in pets comes from an article by David Bennett and Christopher May, "Joint Diseases of Dogs and Cats," published in *Textbook of Veterinary Internal Medicine*: "Blanket therapy with anti-inflammatory drugs is a poor substitute for a well-designed program of management."

Drugs, including over-the-counter human antiarthritis medications and analgesics, should never be used in your pet without a doctor's supervision, because many of these products can be fatal in pets. For example, acetaminophen (Tylenol) is often used indiscriminately by owners to help pets with arthritis. In dogs and especially cats, acetaminophen can be extremely toxic, causing liver and/or kidney failure, and can even be fatal. Additionally, while acetaminophen is a good analgesic (painkiller) and helps control fever, it is not a true anti-inflammatory drug. Even though some dogs may receive a bit of pain relief with this drug, it is not the best choice for the treatment of arthritis.

Other NSAIDs, such as naproxen, are extremely toxic and can cause severe symptoms, even death. While I often use an NSAID such as piroxicam in pets with severe pain or cancer, I am careful to monitor these pets and choose other therapies when appropriate. I prefer to first use medications approved for pets, when indicated, according to the guidelines I have given in this chapter.

> *If your pet acts sick while taking any NSAID, stop the medication and contact your veterinarian at once.*

Doctors who prescribe potent nonsteroidal therapy may also prescribe other drugs in an attempt to decrease the possibility of gastrointestinal ulceration and perforation. The one drug shown to be effective in reducing the incidence of gastrointestinal bleeding and ulcers is misoprostol (Cytotec). Another drug, cimetidine

SAFE USE OF NSAIDs IN ARTHRITIC PETS

- A proper diagnosis is essential before considering chronic therapy with NSAIDs.
- NSAIDs are most safely used on an as-needed basis.
- The lowest effective dose should be given.
- For most pets, other, safer complementary therapies should serve as the basis for long-term pain relief and cartilage healing.
- NSAIDs should be considered for chronic therapy only after all other treatments have failed.
- Pets taking NSAID therapy for chronic arthritis relief must have a physical examination, plus blood and urine testing, done every two to three months to monitor for side effects. This is especially true in geriatric patients (dogs older than six) and all Labrador retrievers.
- If your pet acts sick while taking any NSAID, stop the medication and contact your veterinarian at once.

(Tagamet), designed to reduce gastrointestinal side effects in pets or people taking NSAIDs, and widely prescribed, has not been shown to be effective.

While Cytotec may be necessary for some pets, those of us who prefer holistic therapy do not find particularly appealing the use of multiple drugs to help control the pain and inflammation of arthritis. Aversion to using multiple drugs also makes natural therapies (the subject of the next chapter) particularly attractive to pet owners.

Finally, what is the "right" dose of a corticosteroid or NSAID for an arthritic pet? The answer is always: the lowest dose that keeps the pet comfortable. When treated simultaneously with natural therapies, most pets can receive well below the label dosage of pain medication, if and when medications are needed.

SURGERY

Most people don't think of surgery as a potential cure for osteoarthritis, since surgery can't really cure it. Sometimes, however, surgery can prevent osteoarthritis by fixing unstable joints before they become arthritic.

When Fritz, an energetic six-month-old male golden retriever puppy, was anesthetized for surgery to neuter him, I evaluated his hip joints in two ways. First, I physically attempted to pop his hips out of joint. In dogs with normal hips, this is impossible to do. In Fritz, however, the hips readily popped out of joint. (Don't worry! As I mentioned earlier, the procedure is not painful, and the hips readily pop back into their sockets after evaluation.) At this time, we also radiographed his hips. This too must be done under sedation to allow full extension of the legs; otherwise the test is not truly valid. Because the signs that Fritz did have hip dysplasia were clear, and because of his youth, he was a perfect candidate for a total hip replacement. After surgery, he took short-term nonsteroidal anti-inflammatory medications to relieve postoperative pain, and nutritional supplements to help his hips heal with minimal pain and inflammation and to allow the cartilage to regenerate. Fritz recovered quickly from his hip surgery, and he should be able to lead a full life and never develop arthritis of the hips as he gets older.

In young dogs like Fritz, early diagnosis and surgical intervention can resolve the problem long before the joint becomes arthritic. In an older pet recently diagnosed with hip dysplasia as a cause of lameness, total hip replacement surgery often cures the problem.

Another example in which surgery prevents osteoarthritis is the dog with a damaged cruciate ligament of the knee. This crisscrossed ligament is easily torn in active dogs and people. Corrective surgery, in both pets and people, often prevents the arthritis that otherwise would inevitably occur. In my holistic practice, however, I've found that most pets with cruciate ligament injuries respond to aggressive therapy with nutritional supplements, herbs, homeopathics, and laser therapy, and as a result, avoid surgery. Owners of pets with problems that can be corrected or prevented surgically should seriously consider this alternative. Supplements can be used to aid healing without side effects.

I often see pets with severe osteoarthritis accompanying hip dysplasia. In some of these cases, immediate surgery, though desirable, is not an option. Some of these pets are too small to undergo a total hip replacement. In other instances, owners must delay the surgery until they an afford it. For these pets, holistic care — including nutritional therapy, acupuncture, laser treatment, and/or homeopathy and/or homotoxicology is beneficial while they await a surgical cure.

DIETARY THERAPY

As an aspect of treating arthritis, dietary therapy is often overlooked. Changing a pet's diet will not cure its arthritis, but there are some important points to consider regarding diet and the treatment of arthritis.

First, obesity is the most common nutritional disease in our pets. Overweight arthritic dogs and cats bear much greater stress on already damaged joints, so weight reduction is essential for these pets. Switching to a "lite" diet, however, is not usually adequate. "Lite" diets are *not* meant for weight reduction, but instead are designed to decrease a pet's chances of gaining weight (or regaining weight, after a successful weight-reduction program). For an overweight pet to lose weight, he must receive a medically controlled "obesity reduction" diet.

If obesity is not controlled in the arthritic pet, whatever therapy is chosen will be incomplete and possibly futile. Because a pet's obesity has several possible causes, and because obesity may be associated with various serious medical conditions, an obese pet should undergo a thorough diagnostic evaluation, including blood and urine tests. Pets with underlying medical problems, such as hypothyroidism, will not lose weight unless the medical problems are addressed.

Second, part of the holistic approach to pet care concerns proper diet. There are inherent problems with generic, low-cost pet foods. Premium foods are much better, and homemade diets are probably the most nutritious. Nutrients can be lost during processing, so additional supplementation is often advised. Proper nutrition is important to help pets heal, including pets with arthritis.

Third, certain diets contain therapeutic amounts of omega fatty acids and other nutrients. Even if a pet doesn't respond to supplementation with such nutrients, a special diet may benefit the pet. Your veterinarian can prescribe one of these diets if it is necessary.

Now for the bad news. I am not a fan of the medicated and prescription-type diets currently available, because they are not natural or holistic. I prefer to have pets eat natural processed foods or homemade diets, free of by-products and chemicals, rather than these processed foods with various supplements added. In my opinion, simply giving pets a natural diet and specific supplements prescribed for their needs is the best way to go.

At the time of this writing, there are only a few natural foods available that are specially formulated for overweight pets. Check with your veterinarian to see if he or she recommends one of these weight-control processed natural foods. Readers who prefer to prepare food at home for their overweight pets can find recipes for homemade diets in my award-winning book *Natural Health Bible for Dogs & Cats*.

If a medicated or prescription diet for weight loss is indicated, I use it for a short period of time to enable the pet to lose weight, even though the ones currently on the market do not meet my definition of natural or holistic. Once the pet's ideal weight is achieved, I switch the pet to a natural food.

While weight loss is important for all overweight pets, a very few seem not to lose weight, no matter what I feed them. Before giving up on such pets, I prescribe nutritional weight-loss supplements and sometimes thyroid medication in an attempt to lower their weight while they eat the medically controlled weight-loss diet.

One of my goals is to create my own line of natural, medicated diets for pets. Unfortunately, as of this writing, none of the manufacturers who currently make natural pet foods seem interested, despite the overwhelming need for a dietary line like this.

YOUR HEALING GOALS

The best therapy for pets with osteoarthritis aims to relieve pain and inflammation, heal the destroyed cartilage by supplying it with glycosaminoglycans, and produce minimal or no side effects. Your goals in helping your pet are to relieve its pain, slow down the progression of the arthritis, and if possible, actually help the joint to heal. As I noted earlier, most conventional therapies do a great job of treating inflammation and pain but rarely help the joint to heal, and often they actually cause more cartilage damage over time.

Wouldn't it be great if therapies could relieve the pain and inflammation associated with osteoarthritis without causing the side effects seen with conventional medications? Many natural therapies relieve pain and inflammation, and actually supply nutrients to help the cartilage heal and slow down the destructive forces of nature that act to destroy the injured joint. These ancient and innovative methods are presented in the next chapter.

CHAPTER SUMMARY

- The goal of therapy must be to relieve the pain and help solve the problem with minimal side effects.
- The two most common classes of conventional medications for osteoarthritis are corticosteroids and NSAIDs.
- Corticosteroids and NSAIDs help relieve pain and fight inflammation.
- The side effects of steroids and NSAIDs include gastrointestinal, kidney, liver, immune, neurological, behavioral, and drug interaction problems, plus additional cartilage damage.
- Surgery is an option for preventing osteoarthritis caused by hip dysplasia and cruciate injuries, and total hip replacement surgery can "cure" it.

CHAPTER FIVE

NATURAL THERAPIES *for* ARTHRITIS: NUTRITIONAL *and* CHONDROPROTECTIVE SUPPLEMENTS

AS PEOPLE TURN TO MORE NATURAL, holistic care for their own bodies, many are choosing the same approach for their pets. Treatment modalities for pets with arthritis include nutritional supplements containing glucosamine, chondroitin, and hyaluronic acid, which supply the building blocks for normal cartilage growth and repair. Acupuncture, chiropractic, laser therapy, homotoxicology, and homeopathy also have a place in the treatment of arthritis.

A number of other natural therapies are available, but examining in detail all of these therapies is beyond the scope of this book. I will concentrate on the most popular complementary treatments for the pet with arthritis.

Keep in mind that often several different types of complementary therapies can be used simultaneously in an effort to maximize the chance of a successful outcome. Using multiple products and therapies may also decrease the need for conventional treatments. There's no way I can say what you should use for your pet, since each pet has individual needs. But I can emphasize the holistic approach and suggest that you work with your own veterinarian to determine which course of therapy is best for your pet.

NUTRITIONAL SUPPLEMENTS

A number of nutritional supplements are available that may benefit the pet with arthritis. Some of these supplements include enzymes, green foods, fatty acids, and antioxidants. Some contain glucosamine, chondroitin, and hyaluronic acid, the building blocks of cartilage. Supplements can be useful by themselves or can be used in conjunction with conventional therapies or other natural therapies, depending on each pet's individual needs. The dosages of many pets' nonsteroidal medications can be reduced when the pets are taking nutritional supplements, with the ultimate goal of weaning them off all medications.

Keep in mind that, even with the variety of supplements we have at our disposal, *supplements are not cure-alls*. No one supplement is perfect for every pet in every situation, and there is no single "best" product for helping pets with arthritis. How do you decide which supplement to use? That is not an easy question to answer. Doctors often have a favorite supplement. And if one product doesn't produce the desired effect, your doctor has a choice of other products he or she can try. Unless the product contains drugs or chemical fillers, there are usually no side effects when used as directed. But because the supplement industry is young and not stringently regulated, owners should use these products *only* under veterinary supervision.

> *While you can use many great supplements for treating arthritis in pets, there is no "ideal" supplement, and supplements are not cure-alls.*

Often veterinarians must try several products before they obtain a positive response. Commonly, I use several supplements to get an additive effect — that is, to get the best response, I use more than one therapy at a time. It may take two to three months before you see positive effects from supplements as your dog's body detoxifies and begins assimilating more nutrients.

A good supplement should meet the following criteria:

- The supplement should not harm your pet.
- The supplement should be palatable so that your pet will ingest it.
- The supplement should be easy for you to administer. Many medications prescribed by doctors are never given to the pet because owners experience difficulty giving the dog or cat a pill or liquid. Supplements come as pills, as liquids, as chewable tablets, or as a powder to be sprinkled on the pet's food. The powdered form may be the easiest to give pets. Supplements designed specifically for dogs and cats, not people, may be easier to deal with because manufacturers usually attempt to put them into a palatable form that is easy to administer. This is one of several reasons why I prefer that you use supplements specifically designed for dogs and cats.
- The supplement should not interfere with other therapies that may be necessary for the pet.
- The correct dosage of the supplement should be known. This requirement is the hardest to meet. Many supplements are recommended on anecdotal evidence and clinical experience and are not accompanied by hard scientific studies that establish ideal dosages. This doesn't mean the supplements can't be used effectively. Many supplements for which the "best" dosage is not known are used safely and effectively to treat arthritic dogs. Because

many supplements lack studies that establish their proper use, you must work closely with your doctor to review the information on available supplements to find the most appropriate dosage possible. When supplements fail to work, the simple reason may be that the dosage was incorrect.

- The supplement must be cost-effective. If it costs too much, owners won't buy it. However, owners should keep in mind that, if the supplement can prevent or cure disease, this will save the owner money in veterinary expenses. Paying a little extra for the supplement will be cost-effective over the life of the pet.

On the topic of cost, it is important to pick a supplement that is cost-effective on a per-day or per-dose basis, rather than simply looking at the cost of the bottle. Here's why. Let's suppose you find a bottle of joint supplement at the local pet store or health food store that contains ninety pills and costs $20. And let's say I have a supplement I would like to prescribe for your pet that also contains ninety pills but costs $60. Which is the more cost-effective supplement?

At first glance you may be tempted to choose the $20 supplement, since it seems much cheaper than the $60 one. However, you can't determine the cost without one more piece of information. The correct dosage for this joint supplement is 1,000 mg twice a day. Each pill in the $20 bottle is 250 mg. To obtain that dosage, you would need to give your pet eight pills per day from the $20 bottle you found at the health food store or pet store. This means the bottle of ninety pills will last eleven days.

If you choose the supplement I prescribe, you will give your pet one pill twice daily, since it's a more concentrated product, at 1,000 mg per pill. This $60 bottle will last you forty-five days, making it much less expensive on a per day or per dose basis (more cost-effective) than the other supplement, even though the bottle costs more. To get the best value for your dollar, you must compare the costs on a per day or per dose basis.

Look to see if the manufacturer of the supplement has the National Animal Supplement Council's seal of approval. This designation is voluntary, but it indicates the manufacturer's desire to prove the purity of the ingredients and the product's safety and effectiveness. Many good animal supplements on the market do not have this label, but if you find a product with the seal, you'll know it meets stringent requirements.

When supplements work, they allow you to reduce the dosage of medications that have the potential to cause serious side effects. Holistic doctors, myself included, have no problem trying products based on anecdotal information, but we would like to see additional scientific studies done to determine the true effectiveness of any complementary therapy. I encourage you to talk with your pet's doctor about trying any supplement. While supplements are safe and rarely cause side effects when properly prescribed and used, you want to be sure that the doctor is aware of every aspect of your dog's treatment.

What about the use of "people" supplements for your pet? I'm often asked if it is okay for owners to give their dogs or cats some of their own joint supplements rather than something else that could be purchased for the pets. It is true that the raw ingredients are the same whether the supplement is designed for a person, a dog, or a cat. However, here are some things to keep in mind before giving your supplement to your pet.

1. The dosage is usually different for pets and people, so you will need your veterinarian's advice on how much of your supplement to administer to your dog or cat.

2. Supplements made for people may not be palatable to pets and so may be more challenging to administer.

3. It may be more expensive to administer to your pet a supplement you take.

4. Many manufacturers make supplements for people, and I have devoted time to investigating only a few of these companies. If you choose to administer a supplement to your pet that you take, it is imperative that you do the research to make sure the manufacturer follows good manufacturing practices. There's a lot of junk out there masquerading as high-quality supplements, so do your homework or you will waste your time and money and possibly hurt your pet by administering the wrong supplement.

5. Keep in mind that *natural* does not always mean "safe." There are reports of people and pets being harmed because a supplement they took was the wrong dosage, the supplement interacted with other supplements or conventional medicines, the supplement was composed of the incorrect species of the herb listed on the label, or the supplement's ingredients were contaminated or otherwise adulterated.

Enzymes

Enzymes are used for a variety of functions in the pet's body. Cellular processes, digestion, and absorption of dietary nutrients depend on the proper enzymes. Most commonly, owners think of enzymes as necessary for the digestion of food, and indeed enzymes produced by the pancreas are essential for that. Once properly digested by pancreatic enzymes, dietary nutrients can be absorbed by the pet. The enzymes produced by the pancreas are amylase, lipase, and various proteases. Amylase is used by the body for digesting carbohydrates, lipase is used for digesting fats, and proteases are used for digesting proteins.

Enzymes found in food too contribute to digestion and nutrient absorption. Natural raw diets contain many useful chemicals, including enzymes, not found in processed diets. Food enzymes begin to break down at temperatures between 120 and 160 degrees Fahrenheit, and break down at temperatures below freezing, which means that processing alters pet food by depleting it of important enzymes. Supplements can replenish enzymes absent from processed foods. Even pets on natural raw diets often benefit from additional enzymes, which is why enzymes are often recommended as a supplement for pets on such diets.

> *Nothing is magical about enzymes themselves.*
> *They work by liberating essential nutrients*
> *in the pet's diet.*

While enzymes are typically thought of as essential for digestion and are commonly prescribed for pets with digestive problems, they may also benefit pets with inflammatory conditions, including arthritis. In such cases, enzymes work differently. When we give a pet enzymes on an empty stomach, the enzymes may actually counteract ("digest") the chemicals in the pet's body that degrade cartilage and cause pain and inflammation. The best way to achieve maximum effectiveness from enzyme therapy for inflammatory conditions is to give the enzymes frequently (several times per day) without food (if the pet's stomach is not empty, the enzymes will be used by the body to digest food rather than remove inflammatory chemicals).

Enzyme supplementation is inexpensive, safe, and easy to administer in pill or powder form. Your doctor can help you decide which product is best for your pet's condition.

Fats in the form of fatty acids are commonly used as supplements in both the human and the animal health care fields. Researchers first discovered that fatty acids were helpful in treating some pets that had allergic dermatitis, and fatty acids are now considered an essential part of every pet's diet. Other practitioners have prescribed fatty acids for pets with dry, flaky skin and dull haircoats. Recently, fatty acids have been promoted for use in pets with kidney disease, elevated cholesterol, heart disease, cancer, and arthritis.

When discussing fatty acids, we're not just talking about adding some vegetable oil to the pet's diet to get a nice shiny coat. The fatty acids that most concern us are the omega-3 and omega-6 fatty acids. The omega-3 fatty acids eicosapentaenoic acid, or EPA, and docosahexaenoic acid, or DHA, are derived from the oils of coldwater fish (such as salmon and trout). Alpha-linolenic acid (ALA) is an omega-3 fatty acid found in flaxseed, walnuts, enriched eggs, and green leafy vegetables. Omega-6 fatty acids (linoleic acid, or LA, and gamma-linolenic acid, or GLA) are derived from the oils of seeds, such as evening primrose, black currant, and borage. Omega-9 fatty acids (including the mono-unsaturated fatty acids in olive oil) replace omega-6 fatty acids in cell membranes and lead to increased incorporation of omega-3 fatty acid in the cell membranes, and they are anti-inflammatory.

Often fatty acids are added to the diet along with other supplements to attain an additive effect. This is especially common in arthritic patients, as fatty acid supplements by themselves usually fail to relieve pain and lameness.

Just how do fatty acids work to help control arthritis in pets? Remember that, in my earlier discussion of inflammation, I noted that cell membranes contain phospholipids. When membrane injury occurs, an enzyme acts on the phospholipids in the cell membranes to produce fatty acids, including arachidonic acid (an omega-6 fatty acid) and eicosapentaenoic acid (an omega-3 fatty acid). Further metabolism of the arachidonic acid and eicosapentaenoic acid by additional enzymes (the lipoxygenase and cyclooxygenase pathways) leads to the production of chemicals called eicosanoids. The eicosanoids produced by metabolizing arachidonic acid are pro-inflammatory and cause inflammation, suppress the immune system, and cause platelets to aggregate and clot; the eicosanoids produced by metabolizing eicosapentaenoic acid are noninflammatory, not immunosuppressive, and help inhibit platelets from clotting.

This sounds simple, but there is some overlap and the actual biochemical pathway is a bit more complicated than I have suggested here. For example, one of the by-products of omega-6 fatty acid metabolism is prostaglandin E_I, which is anti-inflammatory. This is one reason why some research has shown that using certain omega-6 fatty acids can also act to limit inflammation. In fact, people and pets need both omega-6 and omega-3 fatty acids in their diets. Unfortunately, many of the diets eaten by people and fed to pets contain an imbalance of omega-3 and omega-6 fatty acids, resulting in a pro-inflammatory state.

Supplementation of the diet with omega-3 fatty acids works in the arachidonic acid cascade. By providing extra amounts of these noninflammatory compounds, we try to overwhelm the body with the production of noninflammatory eicosanoids. In fact, with time (six to twelve months of supplementation) the noninflammatory omega-3 fatty acids are actually incorporated into the cell membranes of the body, resulting in healthier cells that are less likely to produce pro-inflammatory chemicals when the cells are damaged or die.

Therefore, since the same enzymes metabolize both omega-3 and omega-6 fatty acids, and since metabolism of the omega-6 fatty acids tends to cause inflammation (with the exception of prostaglandin E_1 by metabolism of the omega-6 fatty acid DGLA), by supplying a large amount of omega-3 fatty acids, we favor the production of noninflammatory chemicals.

> *Supplementation of the diet with omega-3 fatty acids may relieve inflammation in the arthritic joints.*

Many disorders, including arthritis, result from overproduction of the eicosanoids responsible for producing inflammation. Fatty acid supplementation can be beneficial by regulating the eicosanoid production.

In general, the products of omega-3 (specifically EPA) and one omega-6 fatty acid (DGLA) are less inflammatory than the products of arachidonic acid (another omega-6 fatty acid). By changing dietary fatty acid consumption, we can change eicosanoid production right at the cellular level and try to modify (decrease) inflammation within the body. By providing the proper (anti-inflammatory) fatty acids, we can use fatty acids as an anti-inflammatory substance. However, since the products of omega-6 fatty acid metabolism (specifically, arachidonic acid) are not the sole cause of the inflammation in our pets with osteoarthritis, fatty acid therapy is rarely effective as the sole therapy. It is used as an important adjunct therapy to achieve an additive effect.

Note: Flaxseed oil is a popular source of alpha-linoleic acid (ALA), an omega-3 fatty acid that is ultimately converted to EPA and DHA. However, many species of pets, including dogs and cats, and some people cannot convert ALA to these other, more active noninflammatory omega-3 fatty acids. In one study of people, flaxseed oil was ineffective in reducing symptoms of arthritis or raising levels of EPA and DHA. Because supplementation with EPA and DHA is important, flaxseed oil is not recommended as the sole fatty acid supplement for pets, although flaxseed and flax oil do have important health benefits and can also be given to your pet.

Because of their anti-inflammatory effects, I routinely use large doses — 20 to 30 mg of EPA and DHA (this refers to the amount of EPA and DHA, not the amount of the oil itself) per pound of body weight twice daily — to treat arthritic dogs and cats. This is several times the label dosage of most fish oil supplements, as the label dosage on most products is too low to provide anti-inflammatory effects. Giving arthritic pets fatty acid supplements often allows doctors to lower the dosages of drugs such as corticosteroids and nonsteroidal anti-inflammatory medications, and a recent study showed that dogs taking fish oil did well on reduced dosages of the NSAID carprofen, a reduction that minimized carprofen's potential side effects. Since processed foods contain increased omega-6 fatty acids and decreased omega-3 fatty acids, supplementation with omega-3 fatty acids, especially for the arthritic pet, seems warranted.

Because flaxseed oil contains the omega-3 fatty acid ALA, it is not recommended as the sole fatty acid supplement for pets, since many pets are unable to convert ALA to EPA and DHA.

While many doctors, including myself, use fatty acids to treat a variety of medical problems, there is considerable debate about the use of fatty acids as a treatment for arthritis and other health problems in pets (allergies, heart disease, kidney disease). The debate concerns several areas:

What is the "best" dose to use in the treatment of pets? Research in the treatment of allergies indicates that the label dosage is ineffective; this is also true when using fatty acids to treat pets with arthritis. In people, the dosage that showed effectiveness in the studies I quote here was 1.4 to 2.8 g of GLA per day, or 1.7 g of EPA plus 0.9 g of DHA per day, which is hard for people to obtain from the supplements currently available. If this were shown to be the correct dosage for pets, a 50-pound dog would need to take ten or more fatty acid capsules daily of a typical supplement to obtain a similar dosage, depending on which supplement was used (and there are many choices on the market).

> *Most doctors recommend using at least two to four times the label dosage of fatty acids to maximize the anti-inflammatory action.*

What is the "correct" fatty acid to use? Should we use only omega-3 (EPA and DHA) fatty acids, or combine them with omega-6 (GLA) fatty acids? Is there an "ideal" ratio of omega-6 to omega-3 fatty acids? The ideal dietary ratio seems to be five to one. That is, five parts of omega-6 to one part of omega-3 fatty acids, although this too is debated. Whether or not this "ideal" dietary ratio is ideal for the treatment of arthritis remains to be seen.

Is supplementation with fatty acid capsules or liquids the best approach, or is dietary manipulation (creating a diet that incorporates the "ideal" ratio of omega-6 and omega-3 fatty acids) preferred for the treatment of inflammatory conditions like osteoarthritis? There are in fact diets constructed with this "ideal" ratio. For owners who do not like giving their pets medication, or for pets that don't take the fatty acid supplements easily, it may be wise to try some of these medically formulated diets (available from your pet's doctor) that contain fatty acids. These diets, often prescribed as anti-inflammatory diets for pets with allergies, may be useful as a part of the therapy for arthritic pets. However, I should point out that these diets are typically not the holistic, natural diets that I recommend, and they often contain by-products and chemicals. For this reason, I prefer to supplement a great diet with extra omega-3 fatty acids.

When deciding how much of a fatty-acid product to give your pet, it's important to understand how to read the label. This is an area of much confusion for both pet owners and doctors. Many pet owners and doctors use the fish oil content of the fatty acid supplement as their guideline for dosing. However, this is incorrect. The proper way to dose a fatty acid is to ignore the total fish oil concentration, instead paying attention to the additive effect of the active omega-3 fatty acids, EPA and DHA.

As an example, let's suppose that your pet should take 500 mg of EPA and DHA twice daily. If each capsule contains 250 mg of EPA and DHA, then *regardless of the amount of fish oil in the capsule*, you would give your pet two of these capsules twice daily.

Some fish oil supplements don't list a milligram amount of EPA and DHA, but instead list these amounts as percentages. This is confusing, and it's often difficult for me to figure out how much of the supplement a patient should receive. Try to avoid supplements that list ingredients as a percentage. If you can't do so, you must call the manufacturers and have them convert the percentage to a milligram amount in order to properly figure out dosing.

Health Maintenance Formulas

Many products that contain a variety of ingredients — such as barley grass, wheat, rice, enzymes, fatty acids, vitamins, minerals, seaweed, and alfalfa — claim to be health formulas. We don't really know why these compounds often seem effective in treating pets for arthritis. Obviously, they supply nutrients missing from the dog's diet, most likely antioxidants, vitamins, and minerals. As in the case of fatty acid supplements, it may be that they interfere with the production of pro-inflammatory compounds. Possibly, they also supply nutrients for the chondrocytes, which produce substances that help heal and maintain a normal joint. Because so many different products are available, it would be wise to discuss with your pet's veterinarian whatever products you may discover.

One of my favorite supplements to give my patients to maintain their health, including the health of their joints, is Vim & Vigor by Pet-Togethers, a company that I consult for. It is a unique product available in a flavored chewable tablet for dogs and a bacon-flavored powder for cats. My patients and my own pets love this supplement, which they consider a treat. You can learn more about Vim & Vigor, and order it, at www.pettogethers .net/healthypet.

Antioxidants

Certain vitamins and minerals function in the body to reduce oxidation, a chemical process that occurs in the body's cells. After oxidation occurs, certain by-products, such as peroxides and "free radicals," accumulate. These cellular by-products are toxic to the cells and surrounding tissue. The body removes these by-products by producing additional chemicals called antioxidants, which neutralize the oxidizing chemicals. In disease, excess oxidation can occur, and the body's normal antioxidant abilities become overwhelmed. This is where supplying antioxidants to your pet can help.

You can use any of several antioxidants to supplement treatment of your arthritic pet. Most commonly, we prescribe the antioxidant vitamins A, C, and E, and the minerals selenium, manganese, and zinc. Other antioxidants include superoxide dismutase, glutathione, cysteine, coenzyme Q10, ginkgo biloba, bilberry, grape seed extract, and pycnogenol (an antioxidant that is promoted as an antiarthritis agent in people and that may also be helpful for relieving pain and inflammation in arthritic pets).

Antioxidants work in a variety of ways, but the end result

is the same: they reduce inflammation, usually by inhibiting the prostaglandins that cause inflammation. As is the case with many supplements, there probably is an additive effect when multiple antioxidants are combined.

Can antioxidants such as vitamin C actually prevent arthritis and skeletal problems in pets? Pet owners who want to prevent the common problem of hip dysplasia and secondary osteoarthritis in their puppies frequently ask this question. What does the research show?

Currently, there are two conflicting sources of information dealing with this topic. In the chapter "Developmental Orthopedics: Nutritional Influences in the Dog," in *Textbook of Veterinary Internal Medicine*, Dr. Daniel Richardson cites one study that looks at this issue. Researchers studied eight litters of German shepherd puppies from known dysplastic parents or from dogs that had previously produced puppies with dysplasia. The adult female dogs were given sodium ascorbate daily during pregnancy, and after birth the puppies received sodium ascorbate until they were two years of age. No dysplasia was seen in any of the puppies, although no radiographic (X-rays) studies or long-term follow-up was done. Dr. Richardson, however, concluded that there is no evidence that vitamin C supplementation prevents hip dysplasia. To substantiate this claim, he argues that if vitamin C deficiency causes hip dysplasia, the other joints would not be spared. He also observes that, since dogs make their own vitamin C and so do not have a dietary requirement for it, they cannot develop a deficiency.

Since vitamin C is a safe vitamin, incorporating it into a regimen to help patients with arthritis is not harmful and may help.

Dr. Wendell Belfield presents the other side of the argument in *Complementary and Alternative Veterinary Medicine: Principles and Practice*. Belfield was the source of the study of the eight litters of German shepherd puppies that I just mentioned. He believes that vitamin C can prevent, and treat pets with, hip dysplasia and other joint conditions, including osteochondrosis and osteoarthritis.

What, then, is the truth? I believe that additional controlled studies are needed to determine the effectiveness, if any, of using only antioxidants to prevent and treat joint diseases. Since vitamin C is made by dogs and cats and not required in their diets, it is hard to imagine a true deficiency occurring. Yet it is certainly possible that, while not required in the diet, additional vitamin C may be helpful in healing or preventing joint problems (some of the common chondroprotective joint supplements include added vitamin C for this purpose). While Dr. Belfield's research is impressive, further studies documenting his findings are indicated, including radiographic studies of the pets and long-term follow-up to see if problems develop over the life of the pets. Still, since vitamin C is a safe vitamin, incorporating it into a regimen to help patients with arthritis is not harmful and may help.

CHONDROPROTECTIVE SUPPLEMENTS

When we talk about chondroprotective agents, we're talking about "cartilage-protective" compounds. Unlike corticosteroids and other medications, these products actually help the cartilage rebuild and repair itself. In essence, they are "cartilage-friendly" products. These compounds also help relieve pain and inflammation. Chondroprotective agents can be given orally or by injection, and often both forms can be given simultaneously to the pet that is severely arthritic and in pain. These supplements typically contain one or more of the following ingredients: glucosamine, chondroitin, methylsulfonylmethane (MSM), hyaluronic acid, and various herbs, vitamins, and minerals.

Optimum functioning of the joints is important for pain-free movement. While any pet can exhibit lameness or arthritis, the older pet is more commonly affected. As noted earlier, the articular cartilage (cartilage that lines the joints) must remain healthy to allow the pet to function to maximum capability. The articular cartilage acts as a shock absorber for the joint, providing a smooth surface between bones to eliminate bone-on-bone contact. As the cartilage is destroyed, bony surfaces make contact and irritate each other, causing pain and inflammation and leading to reduced activity. While corticosteroids and certain nonsteroidal medications relieve the pain and inflammation, they further destroy the articular cartilage, making a bad situation even worse.

Cartilage is made of cells called chondrocytes, which make a matrix of molecules that add to the strength of the cartilage. This matrix consists of collagen, a protein that connects tissues, and of substances called proteoglycans. These proteoglycans are made of glycosaminoglycans and hyaluronic acid. Surrounding the cartilage, and bathing the joint, is joint (synovial) fluid. Cartilage is a tough material that protects the underlying bones and acts as a shock absorber for the joints during movement. A certain amount of wear and tear on the joint cartilage is normal. The various cells and fluids are constantly being broken down and synthesized anew. It is important that the cartilage receive proper nutrition, especially when damaged and inflamed. Chondroprotective agents replenish the raw materials that are essential for the healing and synthesis of cartilage, its matrix, and the joint fluid.

Various products, each supplying different nutrients, are available to assist in relieving inflammation and to help damaged cartilage to heal. The following ingredients may be included in nutritional chondroprotective products. Although each doctor has a favorite product, your doctor may suggest trying a different product if one doesn't help your pet. Keep in mind that these products have no harmful side effects like those often encountered with long-term use of corticosteroids or nonsteroidal anti-inflammatory medications.

> *You can choose from many chondroprotective supplements.*
> *If one doesn't help your pet, your doctor may suggest*
> *trying a different product.*

Shark Cartilage

There is reported a link between blood vessel growth and the development of osteoarthritis. In the synovial (joint) fluid of arthritic pets, there is an increasing amount of a chemical called endothelial cell-stimulating angiogenic factor. This chemical encourages the growth of new blood vessels in the arthritic joint. It is theorized that, by inhibiting angiogenesis (new blood vessel growth), we may be able to prevent further degeneration of the cartilage.

In the laboratory, shark cartilage has been shown to contain chemicals that inhibit blood vessel formation. Because arthritis is an inflammatory condition, and inflammation requires blood vessels, it has been suggested that, by inhibiting the formation of new blood vessels, shark cartilage can benefit arthritic pets. And in fact, research has shown this to be the case. In studies of both people and dogs, significant improvement has been seen in patients suffering from arthritis. Arthritic pets and people taking shark cartilage supplements often experience increased mobility and decreased pain. In one study, eight of ten dogs showed improvement (defined as no continuing lameness, a lack of swelling and pain, and improved movement) when treated at a dosage of 750 mg per 5 kg of body weight for three weeks. When treatment was temporarily discontinued, pain and lameness returned. Administering additional shark cartilage at 50 percent of the original dose resulted in improvement. The relief from pain and inflammation was theorized to be a result of decreased blood vessel formation. Relief from pain may also have resulted from the large amount of mucopolysaccharides contained in the shark cartilage, which can help nourish and heal the cartilage of an arthritic patient.

As a result of studies such as this one, many veterinarians feel it is prudent to prescribe shark cartilage, since it can be beneficial to some pets with arthritis and can substitute for therapy with medications like nonsteroidal anti-inflammatory drugs, which have potential side effects. The main problem with using shark cartilage to treat arthritis is the large dosage required. The suggested dosage would require giving a large number of capsules to the pet each day. And since shark cartilage is among the more expensive supplements, the dosage needed for a medium- to large-breed arthritic dog would be unaffordable for most pet owners.

> *Shark cartilage contains chemicals that inhibit blood vessel formation.*

Currently, because of environmental concerns over the killing of sharks, and because of the fact that there are better choices available for joint therapy, most holistic veterinarians do not recommend shark cartilage for their patients.

Bovine Cartilage

Bovine cartilage has proven useful in relieving pain and inflammation in human patients with osteoarthritis and rheumatoid arthritis; increased joint mobility has also been noted. In dogs treated with bovine cartilage, good results have been seen in the treatment of degenerative disk disease and some spinal disorders. The recommended dosage of bovine cartilage is 200 mg per 25 pounds of body weight. Like shark cartilage, bovine cartilage is high in glycosaminoglycans, which can help the body repair damaged joints. Since shark cartilage has been found to be a thousand times more effective in preventing new blood vessel growth, it has, for many doctors, replaced bovine cartilage as a supplement.

Perna Mussels

Perna canaliculus, the green-lipped mussel, is considered an effective anti-inflammatory supplement because it is a natural source of highly concentrated glycosaminoglycans (GAGs), including chondroitin, as well as complex proteins, amino acids, nucleic acids, and naturally chelated minerals, and is an inhibitor of prostaglandin synthesis. The effectiveness of perna supplementation is probably the result of individual ingredients such as GAGs and omega-3 fatty acid extracts (which can inhibit both the LOX and COX pathways).

My introduction to chondroprotective nutritional products was a product containing *Perna canaliculus*. A new client who had recently moved to our area asked whether I could locate a product containing perna that his previous veterinarian had prescribed for Lizzy, his older, arthritic Old English sheepdog. He told me that he was opposed to long-term drug therapy for his pet, and that the perna product worked like a miracle. Without it, Lizzy couldn't even get up, much less walk normally. The perna product was safe, devoid of side effects, and very effective. Without it, he would have opted for euthanasia because of her poor quality of life. I ordered the product for him and also used it on several other dogs, with good results. Perna is inexpensive and readily accepted by most dogs. The recommended dosage is 300 mg per

15 pounds of body weight. While safe, it should not be given to pets with allergies to fish or shellfish.

Sea Cucumber

The sea cucumber *Cucumaria frondosa*, also known by the names "trepang" and "beche de mer," is a marine animal related to urchins. Supplements containing sea cucumbers inhibit harmful prostaglandins that cause pain and arthritis. Specifically, sea cucumber oil contains two anti-inflammatory fractions. One fraction has fatty acid characteristics similar to those of the anti-inflammatory omega-3 fatty acids found in coldwater fish. The other oil fraction is a mixture of branched chain fatty acids, mainly 12-MTA (methyltetradecanoic acid) and 13-MTA, which are potent inhibitors of the 5-LOX (lipoxygenase) enzyme system. These fatty acids are possibly produced by bacteria that live in the sea cucumbers.

These marine animals are also rich in nutrients needed to produce cartilage, including chondroitin and mucopolysaccharides, and several vitamins and minerals (vitamins A and C, riboflavin, niacin, calcium, iron, magnesium, zinc, and sodium).

It has also been shown that sea cucumbers contain saponins (triterpene glycosides), which are similar to the active constituents of ginseng, ganoderma, and other tonic herbs. These saponins exhibit anti-inflammatory properties.

Clinical reports from the veterinary community indicate that most dogs readily accept jerky treats made with sea cucumbers, and that these are highly effective.

Glucosamine and Chondroitin Sulfate

For the treatment of osteoarthritis, glucosamine is the most commonly used chondroprotective supplement, and chondroitin is the second most common. Since significant amounts of glucosamine are not normally found in most diets, supplementation is necessary. Glucosamine supplements may be synthesized or, typically, made from the processed exoskeletons of shellfish.

Glucosamine is an amino sugar that is incorporated into joint cartilage, and it is available as a supplement in one of three forms: glucosamine sulfate, glucosamine hydrochloride, or N-acetyl-glucosamine. Studies show that, while all three forms of glucosamine are effective, glucosamine sulfate seems to be the most effective and therefore the preferred form. This is probably due to the fact that glucosamine sulfate contains sulfur, and sulfur is an essential nutrient for joint tissue. It is speculated that the sulfur portion of glucosamine sulfate, rather than the glucosamine portion, may be more important for joint health.

Glucosamine has several actions that make it an effective joint supplement. It activates chondrocytes (cartilage cells) via modulation of a chemical called interleukin-1. It also stimulates the production of proteoglycans, glycosaminoglycans, collagen, and the synovial production of hyaluronic acid, the joint lubricant. Glucosamine sulfate increases serum sulfur concentrations, which further facilitates the production of cartilage, in addition to inhibiting several enzymes that destroy cartilage, such as serine proteases, collagenases, superoxide radicals, and phospholipase A2. And glucosamine sulfate exerts an anti-inflammatory effect by a mechanism that is different from the synthesis of prostaglandins, most likely by inhibiting the nuclear factor kappa B pathway.

A number of studies in people and pets show that glucosamine is equally effective for treating osteoarthritis when compared to NSAIDs, and it does so without the side effects. There have been a few rare reports of people questioning the effectiveness of glucosamine for relieving their joint pain. Careful evaluation of these negative reports indicated that many of the participants were also allowed to take acetaminophen along with the glucosamine supplement. It was proposed that acetaminophen in some way prevented the participants from receiving the full benefit of the glucosamine supplements they had been administered. Because these rare reports are contradicted by the large volume of reports showing glucosamine's effectiveness, it is likely that study design or some other factor, such as the coadministration of acetaminophen or other NSAIDs, reduced the effectiveness of glucosamine. By and large, research, including clinical studies and clinical experience from millions of people and pets using glucosamine supplements, shows the extreme effectiveness of the supplements in relieving pain and inflammation, and in helping to rebuild damaged cartilage.

Glucosamine is very safe with no side effects; mild gastrointestinal upset is rarely observed; taking glucosamine with food may reduce or eliminate gastrointestinal upset. Since commercial glucosamine supplements are often made from the chitin of shellfish, pets with known or suspected seafood allergies probably should avoid glucosamine supplements, although this may be more a theoretical concern than a practical one. While there have been some concerns about pets with diabetes using glucosamine supplements (glucosamine is made from glucose), there are no reports of pets developing diabetes after taking recommended amounts of glucosamine. In my practice, none of my diabetic patients have had their disease exacerbated while taking glucosamine supplements. Additionally, studies in people provide significant evidence that oral glucosamine taken at recommended dosages does not interact adversely with insulin or with oral hypoglycemic medications, or result in significant alterations in glucose metabolism in patients with type II diabetes.

People taking diuretics may need to take higher doses of glucosamine supplements to obtain the full therapeutic benefits; this is likely also true in pets.

Dosages vary depending on the product. As a guideline for combination products, a starting dose of 1,000 to 1,500 mg of glucosamine is recommended per day for a dog weighing 50 to 100 pounds. This dose is then lowered after four to eight weeks. For cats, I use about 250 to 500 mg of glucosamine per day per cat.

Chondroitin sulfate is the major glycosaminoglycan found in cartilage and the most abundant GAG in the body. It causes cartilage to absorb water and retain nutrients, enhancing the thickness and elasticity of cartilage. Chondroitin also stimulates chondrocytes to synthesize cartilage, collagen, and proteoglycan production, and it enhances levels of hyaluronic acid. Chondroitin likely helps inhibit enzymes that are destructive to the joint. It may also lower blood cholesterol levels and is often associated with a reduced risk of oxalate stone formation in the urinary bladder. Studies show that it may take two to six months of usage, or longer, to achieve maximum effectiveness, but that the effects of chondroitin sulfate can last for several months after discontinuing its use.

Chondroitin is composed of a protein core linked to GAGs and polysaccharide chains and sulfates. Chondroitin sulfate is normally made by the body and is secreted by chondrocytes, although production tends to decrease with age (which may be part of the reason older people and pets are more likely to develop arthritis). Animal cartilage is the only dietary source of chondroitin, and supplements are prepared from cartilage.

Even though chondroitin sulfate is a large molecule, studies do show it is absorbed by the digestive system. However, high-quality chondroitin supplements with a low molecular weight are preferable because of their superior bioavailability. Chondroitin is often added to supplements containing glucosamine. While significant studies are lacking, many people feel that adding chondroitin to glucosamine enhances the ability of both substances to repair cartilage.

Because chondroitin production by the body decreases with age, supplementation with this compound may be especially helpful for older pets with arthritis.

Chondroitin is a safe supplement, and there are no clinical reports of adverse reactions. However, there are rare reports of gastrointestinal side effects in people, such as diarrhea, constipation, and abdominal pain, and rarely headache has been reported, as well as edema (swelling of the legs and eyelids), heart arrhythmias, and hair loss. In canine experiments, decreased red blood cell counts, white blood cell counts, and platelet counts occurred after thirty days of administration, but such side effects have not typically been reported in clinical practice, and the significance is unknown. In the many years that I have prescribed chondroitin supplements in my practice, I have not seen any adverse effects. Nevertheless, doctors often suggest that human patients avoid chondroitin supplements for short periods before and after surgery, and that patients at high risk of bleeding (hemophiliacs and people taking anticoagulants) avoid them because of the structural similarity between chondroitin and the anticoagulant heparin.

There is evidence to suggest that people and pets with enlarged prostate, prostate cancer, breast cancer, or melanoma should not take chondroitin sulfate because it may increase the growth and spread of these cancers. Other joint supplements, such as those containing glucosamine sulfate or hyaluronic acid, can be used safely in patients with these conditions.

Primary research shows that coadministration of chondroitin sulfate supplements with platinum-based chemotherapy drugs (such as cisplatin) may decrease kidney toxicity from the chemotherapy drugs without decreasing their effectiveness. More research is needed to determine this.

Dosage depends on the product used. In general, the recommended dosage is approximately 800 mg of chondroitin sulfate one to two times daily for dogs 50 pounds and over, and approximately 200 to 400 mg, one to two times daily, for small- and medium-sized dogs and for cats.

USING CHONDROPROTECTIVE SUPPLEMENTS

For maximum success when using chondroprotective supplements, consider the following important points.

THEY ARE SAFE AND EFFECTIVE. They are extremely safe and equally effective when compared to NSAIDs.

THEY ARE LESS COSTLY THAN NSAIDs. Cost may be an issue for some pet owners. The typical daily cost of using a glucosamine and chondroitin supplement is approximately $1.50 per day for a 50-pound dog. This cost can decrease: over time, less is required to produce the same amount of pain relief, so the dosage may be lowered, allowing the owner to use the least amount of supplement to maintain pain relief. The comparable cost of the most popular NSAIDs is approximately $2 to $3 per day for a 50-pound dog. While glucosamine and chondroitin supplements are less expensive, they are, as noted earlier, equally effective and they lack the potential serious side effects of NSAIDs.

THEY ARE MOST EFFECTIVE WHEN USED EARLY. Since these supplements work by acting on living cartilage cells, they are most effective when used early in the course of the disease. This requires adequate and early diagnosis.

A RESPONSE MAY TAKE SEVERAL WEEKS. That's because chondroprotective supplements are not drugs but rather nutritional supplements. During the first four to eight weeks, I prescribe an increased "induction" dosage, and then the dosage is lowered as improvement is seen (although I often see results within one to four weeks). Additional short-term therapy with conventional and natural treatments can be used during the induction phase.

THEY CAN BE EFFECTIVE WHEN GIVEN BEFORE SIGNS OF DISEASE APPEAR. Supplements can also be effective when disease exists and no clinical signs are present. In my practice, many dogs are diagnosed with hip dysplasia via screening radiographs and are started on the supplements pending the need for surgical correction, or until clinical signs occur.

PURITY OF THE PRODUCTS IS IMPORTANT. Many generic products that sell for much less than patented products do not have the same quality. Studies that have shown the effectiveness of these compounds have used pure grades of the products. Products of lesser purity, while they often cost less, may also be less effective. Unlike drugs, these compounds are not regulated, and labeling can be inaccurate or misleading. Manufacturers are not required to analyze their products regarding purity, uniformity, or content. Purchase only high-quality products from reputable manufacturers, as recommended by your doctor.

REEVALUATE DIAGNOSIS IF IMPROVEMENT ISN'T APPARENT. Because chondroprotective supplements are so effective in improving symptoms in arthritic pets after four to eight weeks, the diagnosis should be reevaluated after this period of time if improvement is not seen.

GLYCOSAMINOGLYCANS (GAGs): A CLOSER LOOK

I've already talked at length about glucosamine and chondroitin, which constitute the major GAGs in the joint cartilage. Remember that glycosaminoglycans are a major component of articular cartilage.

Glycosaminoglycans function by decreasing the presence of harmful pro-inflammatory prostaglandins and other inflammatory enzymes that degrade the cartilage matrix. This results in reduced pain and inflammation, decreased enzymatic destruction of the cartilage, and stimulation of anabolic (cartilage-building) pathways. The GAGs also appear to increase the synthesis of proteoglycans, hyaluronic acid (a joint lubricant), and collagen.

One novel product called Adequan contains GAGs extracted from bovine cartilage and is available in an injectable form. The recommended regimen is a series of eight injections, two each week for four weeks. If the pet has responded favorably during the four-week trial, we then give the pet an injection as needed (usually one injection every one to twelve months, varying from pet to pet). This injectable product can be used with oral chondroprotective supplements as well. The injectable product can be used to get a faster response than the oral supplements can. Further injections are given as needed, or pets can be maintained on oral supplements according to the response seen and the convenience for the pet owner.

Note: This product has also shown effectiveness when flushed into joints during joint surgery, allowing faster and smoother recovery, according to the *Journal of the American Holistic Veterinary Medical Association* (August–October 1996). Side effects with GAGs are extremely rare, though dose-dependent inhibition of blood clotting has been reported. Concerned owners may want to have their pets' doctors regularly monitor blood coagulation parameters and use homeopathic remedies to help increase blood-clotting factors. Adequan must be used under close supervision if the pet has liver or kidney disease.

HYALURONIC ACID

Hyaluronic acid, or hyaluronan, is another supplement often used to help pets with arthritis. It is so effective that I often use it when other joint supplements fail to work.

Hyaluronic acid's proposed mechanisms of action are as follows. First, it reduces swelling at the site of injury by decreasing white-blood-cell migration and infiltration into the affected tissue. It does this by binding to the CD44 binding site on the white blood cells. If there is enough hyaluronic acid available to bind to most of the CD44 sites on the cells, fewer white blood cells will get to the site of trauma, resulting in less swelling and pain. Second, hyaluronic acid inhibits the arachidonic acid pathway. Bradykinin is produced when serine proteases (tissue kallikreins) cleave high- and low-molecular-weight kininogens. Hyaluronic acid blocks the serine protease activity so that lysyl bradykinin, bradykinin, and arachidonic acid cannot be produced, resulting in decreased pain.

There are two great commercially available hyaluronic acid products for dogs and cats that I regularly use in my practice, and which are made by MVP Laboratories: Cholodin Flex (a chewable treat with choline, which decreases a pet's chances of developing cognitive disorder), and Cholo Gel (a potent gel form that I tend to use for pets that don't like the Cholodin Flex treat or have a more severe case of arthritis). See appendix 1 (page 185) for the results of a study I conducted on these products.

ADDITIONAL SUPPLEMENTS

The following items are frequently also included in chondroprotective products.

Bromelain

An enzyme found in pineapple, bromelain provides additional anti-inflammatory relief by stimulating the good, protective prostaglandins.

Skullcap and Mullein

Skullcap and mullein are natural pain relievers. While not always necessary, these agents may help make the pet more comfortable and may prevent the need for additional conventional analgesics (painkillers).

Yucca

Pets with arthritis often respond well to supplementation with yucca, an anti-inflammatory. Some doctors have reported that in some patients a point of tolerance may be reached at which good results from yucca are no longer obtained. In the laboratory, the yucca plant has been shown to contain chemicals that can be converted into steroids, although it is not known if this also occurs in the body.

USING SUPPLEMENTS FOR DOGS AND CATS WITH ARTHRITIS

Here's my general protocol for using supplements in dogs and cats with arthritis:

- Make sure the pet is eating a good diet.
- Add natural vitamins and minerals to the diet. Use a health maintenance formula (my favorite is Vim & Vigor by Pet-Togethers, www.pettogethers.net/healthypet). This forms the basis for all of our supplementation. Other products I use include Canine Plus, Ligaplex, and Catalyn.
- Add omega-3 fatty acids in the form of fish oil (not flaxseed oil) to give anti-inflammatory relief.

- Use a joint supplement containing glucosamine and/or chondroitin, or hyaluronic acid.
- Depending upon the pet's response, I may add herbs, homeopathic remedies, acupuncture, laser treatment, and occasionally an NSAID for short-term use, if needed.

DMG

Dimethylglycine, or DMG, is formed in the body when the amino acid glycine attaches to two methyl groups (a carbon atom attached to three hydrogen atoms). DMG is found in low levels in foods, including meats, seeds, and grains. Both people and pets make it from choline and trimethylglycine (betaine). Trimethyl-glycine is basically the amino acid glycine attached to three methyl groups. Simply, it has one more methyl group than DMG has.

DMG functions as a methyl donor (a methyl donor is any substance that can transfer a methyl group to another substance). By donating a methyl group, DMG acts as a building block for the synthesis of many important compounds, including choline, SAMe, methionine, hormones, nerve transmitters, and even DNA. DMG also improves oxygen utilization, cellular detoxification, cell protection, and modulation of the immune system, and it enhances the healing process. In addition, DMG functions as a adaptogen that helps maintain homeostasis.

As people and pets age, their ability to methylate declines, contributing to various degenerative problems, including arthritis and cancer. Supplementation for older people and pets may be helpful in reducing chronic degenerative disorders. It is also used as an adjunct treatment for epilepsy in people and dogs.

DMG is extremely safe. The body converts it into its metabolites, which are either used or excreted from the body. It has been recommended for use in pets with a variety of conditions, including osteoarthritis, at a dose of 50 to 250 mg per day. It treats osteoarthritis by acting as an anti-inflammatory. Research indicates that DMG reduces the incidence of arthritis and allows for the reversal of the inflammatory condition of some experimental animals with arthritis. Many doctors prescribe it for horses, dogs, and cats to improve performance and enhance recovery from various health problems. DMG is also considered an antistress nutrient.

MSM

Methylsulfonylmethane (MSM) is a natural anti-inflammatory and analgesic. It is a stable metabolite of DMSO (dimethylsulfoxide). MSM supplies sulfur to the body, which can be used for the treatment of a variety of disorders, including osteoarthritis, allergies, and digestive disorders. For example, sulfur is an essential chemical needed for the synthesis of cartilage, which helps explain its use in the treatment of arthritis. In arthritic cartilage, the concentration of sulfur is about one-third the level found in normal cartilage.

MSM is found naturally in a variety of foods, including meat, fish, eggs, poultry, milk, and in smaller amounts, in vegetables, legumes, and fruits. Because of mineral depletion in farm soil, and because MSM is lost during the storage and preparation of food, some concern exists that dietary sources may not provide enough sulfur to our pets. Additionally, the amount of MSM in the body decreases with age, indicating a possible need for this compound in older pets.

Studies in people and animals show improved joint flexibility, reduced stiffness and swelling, and reduced pain after treatment with MSM. Animals with rheumatoid arthritis that were given MSM showed no cartilage degradation.

MSM appears to benefit pets; more research is needed to determine the optimum dosage and treatment schedule, however.

A suggested starting dosage is 500 mg per 25 pounds of body weight, one to two times daily. MSM is considered very safe; the lethal dose in mice is an amount greater than 20 g per kg of body weight. No long-term side effects were seen when human volunteers were given MSM for up to six months.

> *Animals with rheumatoid arthritis that were given MSM showed no cartilage degeneration.*

CM

Found in fish oils, dairy butter, and animal fat, cetyl myristoleate (CM) is an ester of a common fatty acid (myristoleic acid). CM's action mechanism is unknown but may be similar to that of omega-3 fatty acids (its effects often appear more quickly and last longer than when fatty acids supplements are used by themselves, however). Some doctors have proposed that CM can reprogram certain types of white blood cells (memory T-cells); others suggest that CM normalizes hyperimmune responses by the body and that CM may also function as a joint lubricant and an anti-inflammatory.

A major, multicenter study involving people with rheumatoid arthritis showed significant improvement in 63.3 percent of patients using CM alone and 87 percent improvement in patients using CM and glucosamine together. No adverse reactions were seen, except for mild gastrointestinal symptoms in five patients (the same signs were seen in three patients receiving a placebo).

Veterinarians using a product called Myristin in combination with Myrist-Aid or Myristin Special Canine Joint Formula (which contains glucosamine, MSM, herbs, and antioxidants) have reported success in dogs and cats with osteoarthritis. Improvement is usually seen within two to four weeks of starting Myristin.

It appears that CM may successfully treat many pets with

arthritis without side effects; more studies are recommended. A suggested starting dosage is 100 mg per 25 to 50 pounds, one to two times daily.

SAMe

This abbreviation stands for S-adenosylmethionine, a compound closely related to the ATP molecule that the body uses for energy for the cells. When ATP combines with the amino acid methionine, it forms S-adenosylmethionine. While SAMe has been used in people as an antidepressant, it has also drawn attention as a possible antiarthritic supplement.

One double-blind, placebo-controlled study showed that, in people SAMe was more effective at relieving pain than the placebo and as effective as the NSAID naproxen. In this study, naproxen worked faster than SAMe, however, which took four weeks to achieve its effect. At the end of the study, both treatments produced positive benefit, but naproxen produced more side effects, namely, gastrointestinal distress (a common side effect of potent NSAIDs such as naproxen). Another, similar study comparing SAMe to the potent NSAID piroxicam produced similar results and showed that SAMe had positive effects.

Exactly how SAMe is effective when treating osteoarthritis is unclear, but some theories have been offered. SAMe does show anti-inflammatory and pain-relieving properties. Additionally, laboratory research in the test tube suggests that SAMe may work like glycosaminoglycans (such as glucosamine and chondroitin), by stimulating cartilage cells to produce more proteoglycans. This research suggests that SAMe may help heal the joints as well as relieve pain and inflammation. In one study of rabbits, in which surgery was performed on the joints in an attempt to cause arthritis, the SAMe-treated rabbits showed protection against the development of arthritis when compared to control animals. The treated rabbits had thicker cartilage, more joint cartilage cells, and higher proteoglycan levels.

SAMe shows anti-inflammatory and pain-relieving properties, protects the stomach lining, and may improve the mood of pets with arthritis. But while SAMe shows promise as a treatment for osteoarthritis, it does not appear effective for other forms of arthritis, such as rheumatoid arthritis. SAMe also has some positive side effects in people. It appears effective as an antidepressant, protects the lining of the stomach, and protects the liver against various toxins. Current evidence suggests its toxicity is as close to zero as possible, making SAMe much safer than any drug currently used to treat arthritis.

Unfortunately, there is scant information about whether SAMe is beneficial in dogs. The recommended human dosages range from 600 to 1,600 mg per day, but there are no published veterinary doses as of this writing. Additionally, the cost of SAMe is quite high (several hundred dollars a month for the typical human dose). Although SAMe remains a possible supplement for use in pets, more research is needed, and at this time the cost is prohibitive for most owners.

CHAPTER SUMMARY

- As in the case of conventional therapies, a proper diagnosis must be made before using complementary treatments on pets with osteoarthritis.
- Complementary supplements include nutritional supplements such as natural vitamins and minerals; chondroprotective, or cartilage protective, products; raw foods; and herbs.
- Supplements can be used simultaneously with conventional treatments or other complementary therapies.

CHAPTER SIX

ADDITIONAL COMPLEMENTARY THERAPIES

Herbs are often used in the treatment of osteoarthritis in dogs and cats. While many different herbs are discussed here, it's important to work with your veterinarian to determine which herbal therapies are most appropriate for your pet. Acupuncture, chiropractic therapy, magnetic therapy, homeopathy, homotoxicology, and autologous stem cells can also be helpful, and this chapter examines each of those modalities in detail.

HERBAL TREATMENTS

When an herb is prescribed for a pet, it may be the whole herb or just the active ingredient in the herb. Herbal products too may include the whole herb or just a part of it. When only the active ingredient is used, the other parts of the herb (toxins or other ingredients that may make the active ingredient less effective) are excluded. But some of these excluded parts might otherwise beneficially act in conjunction with the active ingredient. Whether it is better to use whole herbs or just the active ingredients is up for debate.

Many companies make herbs for the human and pet markets, and standard quality controls such as those that exist for pharmaceuticals are absent from the supplement market. Studies have shown that some products have more or less of the active ingredient than is stated on the bottle (and sometimes even none!). And problems have surfaced at times in the human market for herbs, when several products containing Chinese herbs were discovered to be contaminated with various toxins. For this reason, use only products from high-quality, reputable companies. The least-expensive generic supplements are likely to be the lowest quality and of questionable value. In my practice, I use only herbs from companies who have a quality control process that I feel most comfortable with.

Herbs are usually supplied in powder, capsule, or tincture form. Many products made for humans can be used in pets. Unfortunately, the correct dosage for pets has not been determined for many herbs, so veterinarians often rely on clinical experience and extrapolation from human data. The following guidelines serve as a starting point for herbal therapy.

WESTERN HERBS

FOR DOGS:

Give one 100-mg capsule per 25 pounds, two to three times daily.

Give ¼ to ½ tsp. of powder per 25 pounds, two to three times daily.

Give 5 to 10 drops of tincture per 25 pounds, two to three times daily.

FOR CATS:

Give one 100-mg capsule per 10 pounds, two to three times daily.

Give ¼ to ½ tsp. of powder per 10 pounds, two to three times
daily.
Give 5 to 10 drops of tincture per 10 pounds, two to three
times daily.

CHINESE HERBS

FOR DOGS:

Give ⅛ to ¼ tsp. per 10 pounds, two to three times daily.

Give 1 capsule per 20 to 50 pounds, two to three times daily.

Give 5 to 10 drops of tincture per 25 pounds, two to three
times daily.

FOR CATS:

Give ⅛ to ¼ tsp. per 10 pounds, two to three times daily.

Give ¼ to ½ capsule per 10 pounds, two to three times daily.

Give 5 to 10 drops of tincture per 10 pounds, two to three
times daily.

Alternatively, some herbalists suggest using the recommended
dosage for people and adapting it for the pet. Most human
dosages are based on an "average" adult weight of 150 pounds.
So if five capsules per day are recommended for a 150-pound person, a 30-pound dog would receive one-fifth of that, or one capsule. Always start at the lower end of the recommended dosage
for people and then slowly increase the amount given to determine the most effective dose (this is best done under veterinary
supervision).

A variety of herbs are available for treating the dog with osteoarthritis. The study of herbal therapy can be divided into Western
herbal therapy and Traditional Chinese Medicine (TCM). Similar
(and often the same) herbs are used by both schools. There are two
main differences between the Western approach and TCM:

DIAGNOSIS. In Western herbal therapy, a conventional diagnosis is made — for example, your doctor diagnoses osteoarthritis. In TCM, a diagnosis typical of the Eastern philosophy may be made — for example, the pet with arthritis may be diagnosed as having a Wandering Bi syndrome and exhibit a need for strengthening the kidney yang. It is not very important which diagnosis is made, as the herbal therapy would be similar in both cases. The important point is that the proper diagnosis is made by the doctor before beginning therapy.

HERBS USED. Another difference is in the herbs used in each approach. In the Western philosophy, herbs such as willow bark or devil's claw may be recommended. In TCM, a combination of herbs with Chinese names such as du huo or tang kuei may be prescribed, although in the United States the Chinese herbs have Western names as well. What name is used is not important as long as the correct herb or herbal combination is chosen.

While herbal therapy may be effective in pets with arthritis, more research is needed to find the "best" herb or herbal combination and the most useful dosages.

Unfortunately, few studies have been done on the use of herbs for treating arthritis in pets, so most of our information is extrapolated from human studies and from clinical experience in pets. Since so many other natural therapies are highly effective in treating osteoarthritis in pets, herbs are not used as frequently. Still, should you wish to use them for treating your dog, or to hear about the use of herbs for various conditions in pets, it is important to become familiar with what is known about the herb treatment of arthritic pets.

Alfalfa: This herb contains many nutrients and is one of the best herbal therapies for osteoarthritis.

Boswellia: The boswellic acids in this herb are useful for their anti-inflammatory action. One study of people with rheumatoid arthritis found benefit in taking boswellia, and another study found no benefit. The conclusion was that, while boswellia may be helpful, more research is needed.

Capsaicin or cayenne: Capsaicin is the chemical that produces the hot sensation in peppers. It is incorporated into topical creams that are popular with people because capsaicin has been shown to relieve pain when rubbed onto sore joints. In people, the only side effect from topical application is the warm sensation felt when the cream is applied. While capsaicin may be effective, these creams are unlikely to be of much use in pets because of the amount of hair covering the skin. It is also possible that the cream used for people may be too hot for pets and may irritate the skin. Finally, unless the medicated area is bandaged, it is unlikely that the cream would have much contact with the pet's skin, as pets are likely to lick off the cream, especially if any burning sensation is associated with it.

Devil's claw: This herb is used as an analgesic and anti-inflammatory and is often recommended for treating arthritis. Compared with placebo, devil's claw has produced a statistically significant reduction in pain experienced by people with osteoarthritis; no animal studies, however, have been done. The herb appears to be safe for short- and long-term use. Many doctors do not use it in patients with ulcers, since it may irritate the stomach lining, much like NSAIDs.

Feverfew: Because of its anti-inflammatory effects, feverfew is often recommended for the treatment of people with osteoarthritis, and it may also benefit pets with the condition.

Ginger: Considering its ability to dilate blood vessels, ginger may increase blood circulation to arthritic joints.

Horsetail: This herb contains silicon, which serves as the matrix in connective tissue development.

Licorice: Many herbalists regard licorice, a fast-acting anti-inflammatory agent, as "nature's cortisone" and often recommend it for pets with arthritis.

White willow bark: Willow bark contains salicin and is used for pain relief and anti-inflammatory action. The original manufacturers of common aspirin made it by chemically modifying salicin found in willow bark to produce salicylic acid. Willow bark itself can be considered a natural form of aspirin, since salicin is converted by the body to salicylic acid. The side effects associated with chemically produced aspirin can occur in patients given willow bark, so it should not be administered to cats without veterinary supervision (cats are more susceptible to toxicity from salicylic acid than are dogs). However, a very large amount of the herb is required to get the same dose of active ingredient that is found in aspirin. Unlike aspirin, which, chemically, is acetylsalicylic acid, white willow bark lacks an acetyl group. The acetyl group confers an additional property to salicylic acid: the ability to prevent platelets from clotting (antithrombotic effect). This antithrombotic effect is not seen with white willow bark. Salicin is slowly absorbed in the intestines. This means that it takes longer for relief to occur after taking willow bark, but that the effect is longer lasting than that of salicylic acid.

White willow bark was the original source of aspirin.

Common Chinese Herb Formulas

According to Traditional Chinese Medicine, there is no single condition called "osteoarthritis." TCM instead identifies deficiencies or excesses that are found in various body systems, and which create the symptoms Western medicine associates with osteoarthritis. For example, one type of arthritis may exhibit dampness and wind, another might exhibit numbness, and yet another may necessitate tonification of the yin. This means that, when using the Western diagnosis of "osteoarthritis," your pet's doctor may try several herbal formulas before finding the one that works best for your particular pet. A variety of herbal formulas are available for treating pets with arthritis. The ingredients in each formula vary because of the Chinese diagnosis and classification of arthritis. Here are some of the common herbs and the desired result:

Astragalus: Tonifies the qi

Cinnamon bark: Warms the circulation and acts as a spleen tonic

Clematis: Relieves pain caused by wind and dampness and relaxes muscles and tendons

Codonopsis: Warms the circulation and acts as a spleen tonic

Deer antler: Tonifies yang and warms and strengthens the bones

Epimedium: Acts as a liver and kidney tonic

Eucommia: Strengthens the back and acts as a kidney yang tonic

Gentiana: Clears dampness and heat

Ginger: Warms the circulation and acts as a spleen tonic

Hoelen: Drains dampness and acts as a spleen tonic

Licorice: Harmonizes the body and nourishes the supporting structures (tendons and muscles) that can be involved in arthritis

Rehmannia: Nourishes the liver and kidney

Tang kuei: Nourishes the blood and dispels pain

Tuhuo angelica: Nourishes the kidney yang and bladder to expel wind, cold, pain, and dampness; has analgesic and anti-inflammatory properties

White peony: Has analgesic and anti-inflammatory properties and relieves muscle spasms and cramps

Using Herbal Treatments

The use of any of these supplements for the treatment of arthritis does not always yield overnight results. When using supplements, I usually tell owners to give the products at least two months to see if they are effective, although results can be seen in as little as a few days of starting a supplement. Sometimes I prescribe the products at an induction dose (often double the maintenance dose) for four to six weeks, and then, once we see results, I lower the dose to the maintenance dose to decrease the cost to the owner. Some of these products are expensive, especially for larger dogs. While we're waiting to see if we get positive results, the pet may need another form of therapy for immediate pain relief and to control inflammation. Acupuncture, homeopathy, homotoxicology, laser therapy, and even the short-term use of corticosteroids or nonsteroidal anti-inflammatory medications may be helpful.

Occasionally, despite considerable improvement, some dogs and cats may experience a particularly bad day. Medical therapy, laser treatment, acupuncture, homotoxicology, or homeopathy can be useful during these bad days.

Keep in mind that often several different types of products are used simultaneously in an effort to maximize the chance of a successful outcome. Using multiple products may also decrease the need for conventional drug therapy. Work with your pet's doctor to determine which course of therapy is best for your pet.

So, after reviewing all these supplements, which ones should you use for your pet? There's no way for me to answer that, since each pet has individual needs. In chapter 5, I've listed my general protocol for using supplements in dogs and cats with arthritis.

ACUPUNCTURE

Acupuncture is an excellent complementary therapy to relieve the pain and inflammation associated with arthritis. Most dogs tolerate acupuncture well, showing no signs of discomfort; many actually relax or fall asleep during treatment.

I usually combine acupuncture with supplements designed to heal the cartilage, as acupuncture will not do this. Once the pet has improved, I use acupuncture only when the pet shows increased stiffness.

Traditional acupuncture involves the placement of tiny needles into various parts of the pet's body. These needles stimulate acupuncture points that stop the signs of arthritis. After treatment with acupuncture in its purest form, the dog stops limping. Other forms of acupuncture involve laser therapy; aquapuncture, which entails injecting tiny amounts of vitamins at the acupuncture site for a more prolonged effect; and electroacupuncture, in which a small amount of painless electricity stimulates the acupuncture site for a more intense effect.

I choose the acupuncture points after performing diagnostic tests, or according to traditional formulas. These points correspond to areas of the body that contain nerves and blood vessels. Stimulating these points apparently stimulates the release of chemicals — endorphins and enkephalins — in the body. These chemicals, by inhibiting pain, stimulating the immune system, and altering blood vessels, cause a decrease in the clinical signs of arthritis.

As a rule, acupuncture compares favorably with other options for the treatment of arthritis. In some instances, acupuncture may be preferable when conventional therapy is ineffective or potentially harmful (as in the case of corticosteroid drugs used as long-term therapy for pain relief).

Acupuncture is believed to stimulate the release of endorphins and enkephalins in the body.

At other times, acupuncture may be used when an owner cannot afford conventional treatments (such as back surgery for intervertebral disk disease or hip replacement surgery for the pet with severe hip dysplasia). The holistic ideal is that the owner and the doctor discuss both acupuncture and conventional therapies to allow the owner to make the best decision for the dog.

Side effects from acupuncture are rare. However, accidental puncture of a vital organ can occur. Infection can occur at the site of needle insertion. On very rare occasions, the needle can break and surgery may be needed to remove it.

Some pets require sedation in order to allow insertion of the acupuncture needles. In some animals, signs may worsen for a few days before they improve.

Many owners worry that acupuncture is painful and that their pets will suffer. Usually, acupuncture is not painful. Occasionally, the animal will experience some sensation as the needle passes through the skin. Once the needles are in place, most animals relax and some become sleepy.

The number of acupuncture treatments that a pet will require varies from pet to pet. Usually, owners are asked to commit to eight treatments over two to three weeks to assess whether acupuncture will work. On average, treatments last about fifteen to thirty minutes for needle acupuncture and five to ten minutes for aquapuncture or electroacupuncture. If the pet improves, acupuncture is done as needed to control the pet's signs.

Here is an example of a case from my practice where acupuncture worked wonderfully for a pet with hip dysplasia and secondary arthritis. Dusty, a three-year-old Shetland sheepdog (sheltie), was lame. Radiographs (X-rays) taken while Dusty was sedated revealed severe dysplasia of both hips. The hips were easily dislocated while Dusty was sedated. The owner wanted a total hip replacement performed, but the surgeon said that Dusty was too small for this procedure — the implants are made only for medium- to large-sized dogs. The owner considered other surgical options but did not proceed with those. We started Dusty on supplements, including glucosamine, fatty acids, and chondroitin, and began acupuncture treatments twice weekly. After four weeks, we switched from traditional needle acupuncture to electroacupuncture. After eight treatments, Dusty was doing quite well. The owner has maintained Dusty on supplements alone, with the instructions to return as needed for further acupuncture.

Acupuncture points that work well for dogs with hip dysplasia include GB-29, GB-30, and BL-54. Usually, these are the only three points I use. Other points can be selected if the pet does not respond to this particular regimen.

As you can tell, it's vitally important that a correct diagnosis be made *before* acupuncture is attempted. Many owners seem surprised that I stress careful diagnosis, and seem to prefer that I simply grab some needles and start treatment! However, I must first answer these questions: Will acupuncture help this pet? Where do I place the needles? I can't answer these questions without a proper diagnosis. Regardless of whether an owner wants conventional treatment, alternative treatment, or a combination of both, we must have a correct diagnosis. This is yet another good reason to make sure the person performing acupuncture is a veterinarian. Only veterinarians can make a proper diagnosis and prescribe the correct course of therapy.

CHIROPRACTIC THERAPY

Chiropractic medicine is the use of spinal manipulation to improve health. Like other natural therapies, chiropractic medicine is designed to work at the appropriate level of the healing process and to enhance the body's normal, inborn homeostasis (the ability of the body to remain "normal and healthy"), rather than to simply treat symptoms.

Spinal manipulation is an old therapy, almost as old as acupuncture (the Chinese began using acupuncture about 2700 BCE). Even Hippocrates used this discipline, as he felt that the misaligned spine was the cause of many diseases. While chiropractic care has long been used in human medicine, only recently has this discipline been applied to animals. Few controlled studies of animals have shown the benefits of chiropractic therapy, but a number of anecdotal reports have demonstrated positive benefits.

Chiropractic care focuses on the interactions between neurologic mechanisms (the nervous system) and the biomechanics of the vertebrae. In chiropractic theory, disease arises as a result of spinal misalignment that negatively influences the nervous system. Since all body systems are regulated by the nervous system, anything (spinal misalignment being the most common cause) that interferes with nervous impulses to organs could affect the proper functioning of those organs and body systems. Chiropractic therapy is designed to realign the spine by a variety of manipulative techniques.

Spinal misalignment is called a subluxation by chiropractors (this is not to be confused with the term *subluxation*, meaning partial dislocation, as used by conventional doctors). A subluxation is technically defined as a "disrelationship of a vertebral segment in association with contiguous [surrounding] vertebrae resulting in a disturbance of normal biomechanical and neurological function."

Several hypotheses have been proposed to explain how chiropractic subluxations cause disease:

Facilitation: This hypothesis states that the subluxation produces a lower threshold for nerve-firing in the spinal cord. Realigning the spine stops the nerve from firing, relieving signs of disease.

Somatoautonomic dysfunction: This hypothesis purports that the abnormal responses of the autonomic nervous system result from altered nerve function that occurs as a result of subluxations. The abnormal autonomic nervous system may cause disease in tissues regulated by the branch of the nervous system including the heart, digestive tract, and urogenital system.

Nerve compression: This hypothesis states that the vertebral subluxations cause pressure on spinal nerves, which alters the normal transmission in the nervous system. Chiropractors believe that the nerve compression leads to ischemia (reduced blood supply) and edema (swelling caused by a buildup of fluid) of the compressed nerves, which causes the dysfunction.

Compressive myelopathy: According to this hypothesis, vertebral subluxations may compress or irritate the spinal cord, which can cause ischemia and/or edema, leading to clinical signs.

Fixation: The fixation hypothesis of why subluxations cause disease proposes that the diseased vertebrae are "fixed" within their normal biomechanical range of motion; the fixation involves local spinal muscles and nerve receptors.

Vertebrobasilar arterial insufficiency: This hypothesis states that the vertebral arteries are constricted due to the subluxations, which leads to ischemia of the patient's spinal cord or structures of the head.

Axoplasmic aberration: It is purported in this hypothesis that the intracellular movement of proteins, glycoproteins, or neurotransmitters in the nerve cells is altered as a result of subluxations. Accordingly, the altered axoplasmic transport may result in a toxic buildup of proteins, contributing to disease.

Neurodystrophy: This final hypothesis explaining how subluxations of the spine may contribute to disease states that nerve dysfunction is stressful to the body and its organs, and that this lowered tissue resistance can modify the immune system. This hypothesis proposes an interaction between the nervous system and the immune system (such interaction has been demonstrated between the immune system and the neuroendocrine system of the body).

Regardless of which hypotheses may ultimately prove to be the cause of disease resulting from spinal subluxations, chiropractic medicine is intended to "cure" the disease process by correcting these subluxations. Chiropractors correct subluxations by performing clinical examinations and radiographic examinations to determine which vertebrae are misaligned. Once the location of the subluxation has been found, the veterinary chiropractor performing the treatment makes a spinal adjustment. The spinal adjustment, defined as a "specific physical action designed to restore the biomechanics of the vertebral column and indirectly influence neurologic function," is performed as needed to realign the subluxated vertebrae and allow neurologic reprogramming of muscle contractions and healing of damaged ligaments. Usually multiple adjustments are needed, as the body requires time to heal.

Note: Because of the increase in popularity of many complementary treatment techniques, including chiropractic, a number of "animal therapists" have advertised chiropractic care (and massage and acupuncture/acupressure) as part of their "specialty." Only veterinarians, or chiropractors using the technique under direct veterinary supervision, should perform chiropractic therapies on pets. Laypeople should not be allowed to practice any of these medical techniques on pets.

MAGNETIC THERAPY

In recent years, therapy using magnets has gained a following among some doctors and pet owners. It is seen as a safe, simple method of treating various disorders, often producing positive results without side effects or much expense. Does magnetic therapy really work? And if it does, will your dog benefit from magnetic therapy?

Magnetic therapy is by no means "quackish." The earth has a normal magnetic field. The cells in our bodies and pets' bodies also have normal magnetic fields that allow for proper functioning. NASA has determined that rats not provided with a suitable magnetic field in space perish due to disrupted energy flow from altered calcium metabolism. Some doctors attribute many common illnesses to the decline over the centuries in the earth's normal magnetic field.

Doctors theorize that magnets work by means of magnetic lines of force. The strength of the magnetic field is measured in gauss units, and the higher the gauss number, the stronger the magnet. For example, a 1,000-gauss magnet is stronger than a 100-gauss magnet. Magnets are used either as permanent magnets, also called static magnets, or as pulsed electromagnetic field magnets. Static magnets come in bars, beads, or strips. Pulsed electromagnetic field magnets use pulsing current flowing through a wire coil to create a magnetic field around the wire: the greater the amount of current flow, and the greater the number of turns of the wire, the greater the magnetic field that forms. The FDA has approved the latter type of magnet for use in people to treat nonunion fractures, fractures that have failed to heal. Other uses include avascular necrosis of the hip, osteoarthritis, and rotator cuff injuries. No toxic effects have been reported using magnetic therapy.

Magnets increase blood flow to the area, bring in essential nutrients, and help relieve pain and inflammation. Magnets appear to heal the body by removing inflammation and restoring circulation. When blood flow to a diseased site is increased, more nutrients are available for healing. In fracture healing, for example, the use of magnetic fields increases the adherence of calcium ions to the blood clot formed at the site of the break. This allows proper formation of the callus that is necessary for fractures to heal properly.

In the Eastern view of healing, magnets help restore the energy flow of the body to allow healing and proper metabolism. This is similar to one of the theories used to explain the positive effects of acupuncture.

For your pet, magnets may be useful as part of a holistic therapeutic approach for arthritis. They should not be used in acute infectious conditions, on cancerous growths (although some doctors do find them useful in treating cancerous tumors), in acute injuries, in pregnant animals, or in dogs with cardiac pacemakers.

In one study, Dr. Michael Strazza found a reduction of 40 to 50 percent in the healing time of simple fractures by incorporating magnets into the bandage. This means that dogs resumed putting weight on the affected limbs sooner when magnets were used along with conventional fracture repair.

Magnets appear to heal the body by removing inflammation and restoring circulation.

A problem often seen in fracture healing is nonunion of the fracture, in which, as noted earlier, the ends of the fracture fail to heal. In treating more than fifty fracture cases with magnet therapy, Strazza found that no cases of nonunion developed. In two cases of severe nonunion referred to him for evaluation, magnetic therapy allowed healing of the fracture site.

Dr. Strazza also reports success in treating various types of arthritis with magnets. Included in his case studies were dogs with spinal arthritis and paralysis, chronic disk disease, hip dysplasia, and arthritis; older dogs that moved stiffly or slowly; and dogs with stiffness that developed after a morning exercise routine. By using the combination of a magnetic mat for sleeping and a spinning magnetic field, he achieved a positive response in 60 to 70 percent of his cases.

For pet owners who do not want to use a magnetic mat, magnetic collars are also available. The magnatherapy collars use hematite crystals, which are a by-product of iron ore, and can be worn by dogs or cats.

Magnets are not a cure-all for every medical problem. Still they are safe, are reported to be effective as an aid in the treatment of osteoarthritis, and are a relatively inexpensive alternative for pets with chronic arthritis. Magnetic field therapy helps the body to heal by creating a favorable environment for repair. Since specialized magnets are needed for use in therapy, talk with your doctor about her recommendation for a source of the magnets if she feels this therapy may help your pet.

> *Magnets are not a cure-all for every medical problem. Still they are a safe and relatively inexpensive alternative for pets with chronic arthritis.*

HOMEOPATHY

With conventional medicine, we use drugs to reduce symptoms or allow the body to cure the disease. With homeopathy, we use extremely diluted substances to allow the body to cure itself.

First proposed by Dr. Samuel Hahnemann in 1790, homeopathy traces its roots back more than twenty-four hundred years, to the time of Hippocrates. It is based on the law of similars ("like cures like"), the idea that the same substances that, in their full-strength form, can cause a disease may, in a diluted form, cure the disease. The more dilute the homeopathic compound, the stronger it is in the treatment of the disorder.

Homeopathic remedies are prepared as small pills (pellets) with a lactose base, or as a liquid tincture using spring water, with alcohol as a preservative.

If this is the first time you've heard about homeopathy, the concept no doubt sounds strange. As a doctor trained in conventional medicine, I too was overwhelmed when I first heard about the concept of "like curing like." When homeopathic compounds are prepared, often no chemical trace of the original ingredient remains. In effect, it seems like all we're giving the pet is water or lactose, which are the carriers for the original compound. Certainly pets can't get better by simply drinking water or ingesting lactose.

Yet many do get better. No, it's not 100 percent effective in every pet, but homeopathic remedies do work. The idea is that, even though the original substance may be gone because of multiple dilutions, the energy these compounds released when prepared stay in the solution (or pill) and help the pet heal.

> *Homeopathy uses the energy of dilute solutions to help the body heal.*

Skeptics may point to the placebo effect. Certainly, placebo effects are powerful in human medicine. You want to get better, you want the treatment to work, so it works. However, this placebo effect is all but impossible to reproduce or observe in pets.

You can't tell your pet that the homeopathic remedy he's taking will make him stop walking with a limp and then have him just decide to stop limping! Either the treatment works or it fails.

Pet owners attempting homeopathic treatment for the first time must be open-minded and have a lot of faith. Often, because homeopathy sounds bizarre and far-fetched, owners try other therapies first. Only after seeing side effects from drugs and going through all the other options will some owners consent to homeopathy. I understand. I've been there too. When I first started learning about homeopathy, I thought it sounded too good to be true, and certainly it didn't make any sense from a scientific perspective. Yet after trying it a few times and seeing some impressive results, I became convinced that for some pets homeopathy is a viable alternative (or supplement) to conventional therapy.

For those who demand proof of effectiveness, there have been a number of studies (mainly in people) showing positive effects of homeopathy on many conditions, as compared to placebo use. Additionally, laboratory analysis shows specific differences between homeopathic remedies and placebo (plain water or a lactose pill). For example, a study using magnetic resonance imaging (MRI) found distinctive readings of subatomic activity in homeopathic remedies, but did not find this activity in placebo substances.

Additional laboratory studies show that homeopathic dilutions stimulate macrophage (a type of white blood cell) activity and also cause the release of histamine from basophils (a type of white blood cell involved in allergic reactions in people and pets). These results were not duplicated when performed with placebo substances. Both this study and the study using MRI were randomized, double-blind, placebo-controlled studies, the same types of studies used to approve or reject new conventional medications, and which are often called for by skeptics who refuse to acknowledge the possible positive benefits of natural therapies like homeopathy.

Homeopathy has been used effectively for more than two hundred years and has amassed a growing body of evidence-based research. Modern pharmaceuticals have been used for approximately a hundred years (dating to the time of the discovery of aspirin, which was derived from the bark of the white willow tree by the Bayer company).

Finally, to those who suggest that homeopathic remedies can't possibly work because there are no demonstrable chemical molecules of the parent compound remaining in homeopathic remedies, it is worth pointing out that the Food and Drug Administration still considers homeopathic remedies to be official drugs and, as in the case of conventional medications, regulates their manufacturing, labeling, and dispensing. This is something that would not happen if the FDA considered these remedies simply placebos.

One of the nice things about homeopathy is that, compared to conventional medical therapy, it is virtually devoid of *any* side effects when properly prescribed. Contrast this with the large number of prescription drugs that, despite premarket testing, have poor safety records following approval and widespread usage. Homeopathic substances, when properly prescribed, are usually so dilute as to not cause any harm.

> *Studies have shown positive effects in patients treated*
> *with homeopathic remedies when compared*
> *to those treated with placebos.*

My only concern with homeopathy is that pet owners may decide to skip going to a veterinarian for a proper diagnosis and treatment and instead use over-the-counter homeopathic remedies to treat a pet with a serious or life-threatening problem. This would be an ineffective treatment and could result in further illness or even death. One sad case from my own practice drives home this point.

I saw Angel, a ten-year-old spayed female Persian cat for evaluation. Her owner had treated her symptoms of lethargy and lack of appetite with an over-the-counter homeopathic remedy containing a number of ingredients.

Angel had not been to a veterinarian since she was a kitten, as she had become extremely upset and impossible to handle during her visits. She had received absolutely no medical care for nine years and was, of course, an accident waiting to happen.

Because Angel did not improve after taking the remedy for seven days, her owner broke down and brought her in for a visit. The cat did not like her visit, and her behavior limited what I could do for her. However, I was able to quickly perform a physical examination, draw blood, and get a urine sample. The physical examination revealed a very loud heart murmur, indicating heart disease. Blood and urine testing showed severe, chronic end-stage kidney failure. Unfortunately, because Angel's behavior prevented us from doing any kind of treatment for her, and because of her grave prognosis, her owner elected to euthanize her.

By choosing not to bring Angel in at the first signs of illness and instead relying on a remedy that had no chance of helping her severe diseases, Angel's owner unwittingly prolonged her misery. Even though Angel was too far gone and too difficult to treat, many pets can be treated properly if diagnosed early. By delaying proper treatment, owners who elect to treat with over-the-counter homeopathic remedies may do their pets more harm than good. That's why I recommend prompt and correct diagnosis and the use of such remedies for only the most minor clinical signs (mild itching, sneezing, and do on). If a pet with even minor signs does not improve after two to three days of treatment with an over-the-counter remedy, the pet should be properly evaluated.

Over-the-counter homeopathic remedies should be tried only in pets with mild clinical signs for no more than two to three days before you seek assistance from your veterinarian.

Let's take a look at some of the homeopathic therapies indicated for pets with arthritis. One word of caution I'd like to impart before beginning this discussion: Because the less dilute (and therefore weaker) therapies are available for purchase at many health food stores, you may be tempted to try using homeopathy on your own. Before trying any of these therapies on your pet, do see a holistic practitioner and get a diagnosis first. There are several reasons for this:

First, many of the over-the-counter remedies are combination potions rather than pure homeopathic remedies. With homeopathy, it is preferable to use just the one or two remedies that most closely match your pet's constitution and symptoms.

Second, over-the-counter remedies are the least dilute and least potent remedies that can be used to treat your pet. While such remedies are not harmful, they may not be helpful either. The more powerful prescription remedies available from your doctor are more likely to be effective.

Third and most important, not all pets experiencing lameness are necessarily arthritic; serious diseases such as cancer and immune disorders can cause lameness. Failing to seek medical help, and trying home remedies, can be dangerous. While homeopathy can be helpful, you should treat pets homeopathically only under a doctor's supervision.

Before I list some common homeopathic remedies, let me say

that I never use homeopathic remedies without also trying nutritional therapy and supplementation. I believe in treating the pet, not just the disease, which means I like my arthritic patients to be "nutritionally healthy" before we start homeopathy. I feel the homeopathic remedies may work better if we are using nutritional supplements to help reduce inflammation and pain.

There is no one right remedy. A thorough history must be taken and an examination and laboratory tests must be performed to assist the homeopathic veterinarian in selecting the correct remedy or remedies. I have found the following remedies helpful.

Bryonia: For pets whose pain gets worse and worse as they move around. They are often very thirsty, and the least touch pains them, so they snarl or bite.

Calcarea carbonica: This is often needed for overweight, injury-prone dogs. The hips are often affected and are worse during cold, damp weather.

Caulophyllum: The smaller joints (toes, wrist, ankle) are often affected in animals that need this remedy.

Hecla lava: Bony arthritic projections often form in and around joints. Hecla may prevent new bone deposits and even cause the body to dissolve the extra bone.

Pulsatilla: This may help when pains decrease with cold applications and cold weather. Often the stiffness is in the rear legs, and as in the case of those that need Rhus tox, the pains are the worst with first motion. The animals that benefit from this remedy are very friendly animals that are often not very thirsty.

Rhus toxicodendron: These animals are very stiff when they get up, then move more easily as they exercise (like a rusty gate!). Too much exercise can make them stiff again.

Cold and damp makes them worse, and they can be very restless and have trouble settling down.

HOMOTOXICOLOGY

Homotoxicology, developed by Dr. Hans-Heinrich Reckeweg, is very similar to traditional homeopathy, in that both use minute diluted doses of various substances to effect a cure. However, the focus of each is somewhat different. Homeopathy traditionally utilizes a single remedy or dose strategy to effect a cure. This single remedy is chosen for the individual patient and, ideally, is based on study and the absolutely precise determination of individual predispositions to disease states. It requires many years of discipline and study to practice effectively. Homotoxicology, while utilizing the same remedies and dilutions, is based on a "symptom picture," which occurs as a result of many factors and presentations. Homotoxicology preparations typically contain many homeopathic remedies of different concentrations or frequencies. This form of treatment is geared to the underlying body mechanisms that are primarily based in the matrix of the body's tissue (also called the mesenchyme) and that nourish the cells, carry information among cells, and remove the waste products that result from cellular metabolism.

The goal of homotoxicological therapy is to target the cellular and matrix damage and to restore the function of those tissues back to a normal, homeostatic state. Correction of deficiencies and clearing of the accumulated debris and toxins that jam the normal activity of the cells and matrix are the primary aims of homotoxicology.

The large number of homotoxicology remedies offers an abundant source of homeopathic medication capable of effectively promoting the discharge of toxins, cleansing the matrix, activating cell metabolism, and supporting organ regeneration.

The Heel corporation is the exclusive and original manufacturer of homotoxicology remedies. The following are homotoxicology remedies for arthritis.

Bryaconeel: Contains *Aconitum napellus*, *Bryonia alba*, phosphorus

Curoheel: Contains *Hamamelis virginiana*, pulsatilla, *Carbo vegetabilis*, *Apis mellifica*, *Lycopodium clavatum*, Mercurius praecipitatum ruber, silicea

Kalmia compositum: Contains asafoetida, *Kalmia latifolia*, Mercurius praecipitatus ruber

Rhododendroneel: Contains Rhododendron chrysanthum, *Euphorbia cyparissia*, *Spiraea ulmarial*, *Aconitum napellus*, dulcamara, *Ledum palustre*, *Asclepias tuberosa*, *Stellaria media*, benzoicum aciduml, lithium benzoicum, pulsatilla

Traumeel: Contains *Arnica montana*, radix, belladonna, *Calendula officinalis*, chamomilla, millefolium, hepar sulphuris calcareum, *Symphytum officinale*, *Aconitum napellus*, *Bellis perennis*, mercurius solubilis, *Hypericum perforatum*, echinacea, *Echinacea purpurea*, *Hamamelis virginiana*

Zeel: Contains *Arnica montana*, radix, *Rhus toxicodendron*, dulcamara, *Symphytum officinale*, sulphur, *Sanguinaria canadensis*, cartilago suis, embryo suis, funiculus umbilicalis suis, placenta suis, alpha-lipoicum acidum, coenzyme A, nadidum, natrum oxalaceticum

EMERGING NEW THERAPY:
AUTOLOGOUS STEM CELLS

Autologous stem cell therapy, which uses stem cells taken directly from your dog, offers the possibility of an exciting, new, and totally natural therapy for the treatment of the dog with osteoarthritis.

Stem cells are prepared from a small amount of fat taken from your dog while under local or general anesthesia. The fat is sent to Vet-Stem, a company that developed the procedure for harvesting stem cells from fat. After processing your dog's fat sample, Vet-Stem sends the harvested stem cells back to your veterinarian for injection into the arthritic joint(s). Usually, one injection is administered to initiate the healing process. Further treatments are used as needed.

Fat is used as a source of stem cells because there is a high concentration of stem cells in fat, several hundred times more than in the bone marrow.

The cells injected into your dog's arthritic joint contain, in addition to the stem cells, other regenerative cells that produce cytokines (such as interleukin-1 receptor antagonist, which reduces inflammation and fibrosis) and growth factors that relieve pain and inflammation and encourage healing of the damaged cartilage. The injured joint tissues signal the regenerative stem cells as they are grafted into the treated area. Evidence strongly suggests that stem cells turn into tissues similar to the environment in which they are placed.

Because the therapy is totally natural and because the cells are taken directly from your dog's body, side effects are very rare and include those typically associated with anesthesia, minor surgery, and the administration of injectable substances.

Stem cell therapy works by providing a long-term reduction in inflammation; decreasing pain; stimulating the regeneration of cartilage and, in the process, slowing the degenerative processes; and initiating healing in both acute and chronic injuries. It has been proven to work in dogs with arthritis of the elbow and hip joints.

Stem cell therapy can be used in conjunction with most other natural and conventional medical therapies with the following exceptions:

- It is recommended that shockwave therapy not be used following stem cell therapy for at least sixty days because regenerative stem cells require time to reorganize and adhere. Using shockwave therapy prior to stem cell therapy is acceptable and may increase the signaling process and potentially promote the overall healing process.
- Corticosteroids should not be used with stem cell therapy because corticosteroids may adversely affect the harvesting of cells collected for regenerative therapy. Also, they diminish the efficacy of regenerative stem cell therapy once it has been initiated. All therapeutic levels of steroids should be eliminated prior to tissue collection, and the use of steroids should be avoided for a minimum of forty-five days postinjection.
- Therapeutic ultrasound should not be used for forty-five days after implantation, but it may be used before treatment.
- A transcutaneous electrical nerve stimulation (TENS) unit should not be used for forty-five days after implantation, but it may be used before treatment.
- NSAIDs are commonly used to relieve pain and inflammation as part of the therapy for the pet with arthritis. NSAIDs do not interfere with the action of regenerative cell therapy, and their use can be maintained before and after the injection of cells.

CHAPTER SUMMARY

- Herbal therapies help relieve pain and inflammation via the pharmaceutical activities of their ingredients.
- Joint supplements help repair cartilage and reduce pain and inflammation.
- Acupuncture, chiropractic care, and cold lasers relieve

the pain and the signs of osteoarthritis but do not cure the disease.

- Magnetic therapy helps the body to heal by creating a favorable environment for repair.
- Homeopathy and homotoxicology trigger the body's healing response with the help of dilute solutions.
- New therapies such as stem cell treatments offer hope for rebuilding damaged arthritic tissues, but more experience with them is needed before they become standard therapies.

CHAPTER SEVEN

DIET *and* ARTHRITIS

ONE OF THE MOST IMPORTANT FACTORS in your pet's health, and one you can control, is diet. You and you alone control what goes into your pet's mouth. While diet is not the focus of this book, it directly affects pets and influences which diseases they acquire, including arthritis. A more thorough discussion of diet can be found in my book *Natural Health Bible for Dogs & Cats* (Prima Publishing, 2001).

It is important to consider how diet can affect the pet with arthritis. While most doctors and owners neglect the diet's contribution to a pet's health, as well as how a proper diet (especially for overweight pets) can positively affect the pet with arthritis, holistic doctors and owners know that proper diet and nutritional supplementation form the basis of every holistic health plan.

Let's take a look at pet foods first, then we'll talk about obesity and how controlling this major health problem can help the pet with arthritis walk more comfortably.

The main decision facing pet owners is which kind of food to feed pets: a natural diet, whether homemade or processed, or one of the many advertised processed diets available at many stores. Just what constitutes the best or most appropriate diet is a controversial topic, and there are as many opinions as there are doctors, but let's explore this issue for a moment. No matter which type of diet, homemade or processed, is chosen, it must meet at least five requirements:

1. It must contain the proper amount and balance of essential nutrients required by the pet.
2. The ingredients must be of high nutritional quality so that the animal can effectively digest, absorb, and utilize the dietary nutrients.
3. The diet should be palatable so that the pet will eat it.
4. The diet should contain no fillers, such as animal or plant by-products. If by-products are present, as they are in some prescription-type diets for sick pets, the diet should contain the least amount of by-products.
5. The diet should contain no artificial colors, flavors, chemical preservatives, or additives, when possible.

Most processed foods, even "premium diets," contain fillers, by-products, and chemicals that I do not think contribute to health, so my recommendation is to feed the pets most natural and organic diet possible. This diet can be homemade or purchased already made for your pet.

Natural diets differ from most other prepared diets in the following ways:

- They are made of only human-grade, high-quality ingredients. Other prepared diets may use food by-products processed for, but declared "unfit" for use by, humans.
- They incorporate foods, especially grains, in their whole state, rather than parts of those foods (as an example, they include rice rather than rice flour, a rice by-product).

- They include no artificial colors, additives, chemicals, or preservatives.
- They are formulated for optimum nutrition.

As I've already noted, one problem often seen in arthritic pets is obesity. Obesity is a severe and debilitating illness. It is the most common nutritional disease in pets and people; estimates suggest that up to 45 percent of dogs and up to 13 percent of cats are obese (I think these estimates are too low, judging by the number of obese pets I see every day in my practice). Obesity is a disease of domestication. With rare exceptions (such as the presence of a disorder like thyroid disease), obese pets are made obese and not born obese. In the wild, few if any animals are obese. They eat to meet their caloric needs and are always moving, playing, fighting, and hunting for food (exercising). Ideally, you should work with your doctor from the time your pet is young so that you can prevent obesity.

> *Obesity is the most common nutritional disease in pets and people.*

How can you decide if your pet fits the definition of "obese"? Current medical opinion states that a pet is obese if it weighs 15 percent or more over its ideal weight. Pets weighing 1 to 14 percent over their ideal weight are considered overweight but not yet obese.

While 15 percent does not seem like much, consider these figures:

- A Labrador retriever, one of the breeds most commonly afflicted with arthritis, weighing 69 pounds that should weigh 60 pounds is 15 percent overweight and is classified as obese.
- An 11.5-pound cat that should weigh 10 pounds is 15 percent over its ideal weight and is classified as obese.

As you can see, even just a few extra pounds — or less — are cause for concern.

A pet's weight isn't the only way to gauge obesity. I prefer to use body composition. Body composition more accurately reflects obesity and gives us something more concrete to shoot for, rather than some magic number. For example, while most people strive to achieve a certain numerical weight for themselves, it would be better to strive for a certain look. Losing 10 pounds may be an admirable goal, but being able to lose a few inches around the waist or fit into a smaller pair of pants is really the ultimate goal.

I'm not suggesting you can't have a target weight when designing a weight-control program for your pet, only that this magic number is a rough guideline to your pet's best weight as you treat his obesity. Ultimately, I use the look and feel of the pet (measured by the body composition score, which estimates your pet's ideal weight for his skeletal composition) to know when we have reached our ultimate goal. Simply put, your pet is likely overweight if you cannot easily see or feel his ribs or spine. Your veterinarian can assess your pet's body composition during a physical examination.

OBESITY AND ARTHRITIS

Obesity causes problems for the arthritic pet for two reasons. First, the extra weight puts increased stress on already damaged joints. Second, obesity can increase the risk of developing arthritis in the first place and promote a chronic pro-inflammatory condition. In obese people, increased levels of pro-inflammatory chemicals occur, including C-reactive protein, interleukin-6, and plasminogen activator inhibitor. Excess intake of calories may cause oxidative stress to the cells, insulin resistance, and type II diabetes, all of which cause increased concentrations of interleukin-6 and tumor necrosis factor alpha, leading to inflammation and further damage to the joints.

Realize that obesity does not occur overnight, and neither will it go away overnight. While there is a very small subset of pets that truly cannot lose weight, most pets will reach an acceptable weight within six to twelve months of starting an obesity diet coupled with an approved exercise program (see the next chapter). This rate of weight loss approximates 2 percent per week, which is an acceptable amount that will not cause muscle loss. The actual rate of weight loss recommended by your veterinarian may vary according to your pet's needs.

A sensible weight-loss program encourages slow, controlled loss of excessive body fat.

Before starting your pet on a weight-reduction diet and exercise regimen, it is important that your veterinarian conduct a blood profile to rule out diseases we have discussed, such as diabetes and hypothyroidism, that may cause or contribute to obesity. If present, these diseases would require treatment in addition to dietary therapy.

Since various diseases, including diabetes and hypothyroidism, can cause or contribute to obesity, it is imperative to test for them before starting a medically controlled weight-loss program.

If your pet needs to lose weight, ask your veterinarian to recommend a weight-reduction diet. As I noted earlier, store-bought "lite" foods are not designed for weight loss but rather for weight maintenance once weight loss has been achieved. For this reason, they are not usually recommended for pets that need to lose weight. And since most of these diets do not contain natural, healthy ingredients, it is unlikely they could be recommended as part of a weight-loss program anyway, unless other diets could not be used.

Several commercial weight-loss or obesity-reduction diets exist, but many of them contain by-products and artificial ingredients. I prefer to avoid them, but unless owners want to prepare diets for their pets, I use these specialized weight-reduction diets for a few months to help pets lose weight. Once the desired weight loss is achieved, I prefer to switch to more natural and organic diets for long-term feeding.

To conclude, obesity adds to the stress placed on the damaged joints of arthritic pets. This means weight control is an important part of overall therapy for the pet with arthritis.

CHAPTER SUMMARY

- Although diet alone cannot cure arthritis, it can help prevent the disease and ease the symptoms.
- Overly processed packaged foods are the least nutritious for your pet.
- Be aware of additives in processed packaged foods, and read product labels carefully.
- Natural-style packaged foods, whether store-bought or purchased from a veterinarian, are more nutritious.
- Homemade foods can be simple to make and are the most nutritious for your pet.
- Preventing or treating obesity is the most important thing to do for the arthritic pet.
- There is no substitute for a healthy lifestyle as a holistic healing approach.

CHAPTER EIGHT

EXERCISE *and* PHYSICAL THERAPY *for* YOUR PET

ONE OF THE MOST COMMON QUESTIONS I am asked by owners of arthritic pets is: "How much can my dog exercise?" (Exercise is important for cats as well, but since it's harder to get cats to exercise, most of this chapter focuses on dogs, with a brief discussion at the end about how to provide exercise for cats.)

There is no blanket answer concerning exercise and physical therapy for your arthritic pet, but an arthritic dog should exercise enough to benefit its health, and not so much as to further damage joints or cause excess pain. It's important to keep in mind that most arthritic pets can and should exercise. In addition to engaging in good general exercise, arthritic dogs also benefit from specific physical-therapy exercises designed to ease the pain and stiffness that results from their disease.

Arthritic pets can and should exercise.

Dogs are dogs, and you certainly can't keep them in cages forever just to prevent further injury to damaged joints. Studies of people with osteoarthritis have found that controlled physical exercise provides cardiovascular benefits and a positive sense of well-being. The same is most likely true of arthritic pets.

EXERCISE

Exercise increases muscle tone, is good for pets' cardiovascular systems, strengthens owner-animal bonds, and increases the well-being of pets. Since muscles, tendons, and ligaments are so important in protecting joints, maintaining strength and tone in these body parts is important. While various exercise regimens can be prescribed for human patients, most of these are impractical for pets. A moderate exercise program should be initiated under veterinary supervision. Start slowly, and gradually allow your dog to do more as he progresses naturally on his own. If your dog can go only a half mile at a slow pace before experiencing pain, don't push. Let your dog set the guidelines. The exercise should not lead to pain or discomfort. If your dog is sore the next day, skip that day, and then resume at a reduced pace.

> *Exercise increases muscle tone, is good for pets'*
> *cardiovascular systems, strengthens owner-animal bonds,*
> *and increases the well-being of pets.*

For the severely affected pet, nonweight-bearing exercise, such as forced swimming, is ideal, as this strengthens the muscles, ligaments, and tendons while placing no force on the joints themselves. If you can have your dog swim in a pool or tub while supporting the abdomen and chest with a towel sling, this is ideal. Of course, all dogs having access to a pool should be carefully supervised as dogs can and do drown.

Strict rest, including cage confinement, is needed only when acute, painful flare-ups occur. During these days, dogs may benefit from acupuncture, laser treatment, or a dose or two of a nonsteroidal medication. Massage therapy and/or heat is often beneficial on these days as well.

Regardless of which exercise you choose, simply commit yourself to doing it! You may find that you too become more fit from exercising your pet, which is a nice benefit.

While we don't have studies in veterinary medicine that prove the benefits of exercise, as the studies on people do, clinical experience shows that physically fit pets are healthier. And if we want to extrapolate from the literature on humans (as we are often forced to do), the studies are impressive. The January 1996 *Journal of the American Geriatric Society* showed that musculoskeletal injuries rarely occurred during exercise and moderate-intensity exercise did not exacerbate joint problems. And a study in the journal *Arthritis and Rheumatology* showed that physical activity is associated with lower subjective ratings of pain than those that accompany a sedentary lifestyle.

It's good news that a mild exercise program prescribed by your pet's veterinarian can be highly beneficial for your arthritic pet. Since each pet has unique needs and abilities when it comes to exercise, it is important to work with your doctor and communicate how your pet adapts to the prescribed program. The following cases will help illustrate this point.

A mild exercise program prescribed by your pet's veterinarian can be highly beneficial for your arthritic pet.

Pierre, a male yellow Labrador retriever, was two years old when he was admitted to our hospital for neutering. His owner reported no problems with Pierre that would indicate any underlying disorders, but our normal procedure is to do a physical examination before the surgery.

Because all dogs, but especially a larger breed like Pierre, can develop the skeletal problem hip dysplasia, we recommended testing Pierre for hip dysplasia while he was anesthetized for his neutering. His owner agreed with our recommendation, even though she did not expect Pierre to have any skeletal problems; he walked normally and loved to run, jump, and play, and never showed signs of discomfort or lameness.

The hip evaluation is done under anesthesia to allow a proper assessment. In awake pets, it is difficult if not impossible to obtain accurate results. After Pierre was anesthetized, we performed two procedures. First we laid him on his back and extended his rear legs out and away from his body. This positioning allowed us to get perfect pictures of both hip joints. Second, we rolled Pierre onto his right side, and I performed an orthopedic manipulation called an Ortolani maneuver. This maneuver is performed by holding on to the thigh bone (femur) and pushing it toward the dog's spine. In dogs with normal hips, nothing happens, but in dogs with hip joint laxity (looseness), such as occurs in dogs with hip dysplasia, the femur pops out of the joint (resulting in a positive Ortolani sign). In Pierre's case, the right hip joint was normal (negative Ortolani sign). I repeated the procedure on the left hip, which was also normal.

The radiographic (X-ray) findings were quite different, though. Pierre's radiographs showed severe hip dysplasia and severe secondary osteoarthritis in both hips, indicating chronic hip instability caused by hip dysplasia.

Occasionally, tests performed on dogs like Pierre result in contradictory findings: the radiographs lead to one conclusion, and the Ortolani findings lead to another. In these cases, we take the worse signs. In other words, even though Pierre's hip joints were normal during our orthopedic maneuvering, his radiographs still showed severe hip dysplasia. Since it's possible to have contradictory findings in some dogs, it is important to not only take radiographs but also perform orthopedic maneuvers when evaluating dogs for hip dysplasia.

I reviewed the finding of hip dysplasia with Pierre's owner when she came in for his discharge after neutering. I discussed a number of options with her, including surgery to replace the dog's badly damaged hips, medical therapy for pain (as needed if Pierre began to show signs of pain), and nutritional supplementation to help heal the cartilage. Because of the cost of hip joint replacement (approximately thirty-five hundred dollars per hip), Pierre's owner delayed taking this option while she budgeted for the procedure. She elected to correct Pierre's diet, replacing his store-bought food with a more natural processed diet. I also prescribed supplements for Pierre: omega-3 fatty acids and a product containing glucosamine and chondroitin.

Pierre's owner asked about exercising him, because he enjoyed walks, chasing balls, and swimming in the neighborhood lake. Since Pierre was not showing any signs of pain, I told her that exercise would be all right for him. When possible, swimming would produce less stress on the joints than the other forms of exercise would. But since the joints already had significant osteoarthritis, I didn't think those other forms of exercise could make things much worse for Pierre. If he showed discomfort during his exercising, I said, she should cut back on those running and jumping activities that produced direct stress on the joints. Otherwise, Pierre, a very active young retriever, would be difficult to keep quiet and might develop behavioral problems (such as destroying the house and yard!) if he did not have an outlet (such as a controlled exercise program) to expend this energy. At a recheck six months later, Pierre's owner reported that he was doing well and still showing no signs of pain or discomfort from his hip dysplasia and arthritis.

The owner of Bronwyn, another dog I diagnosed with hip dysplasia, was concerned about the dog's level of exercise. Unlike Pierre, Bronwyn occasionally experienced mild discomfort after exercising. According to her owner, this two-year-old female boxer would, from time to time, be a bit sore after playing.

I sedated Bronwyn and took several radiographs of her hips and spine. The films showed very mild hip dysplasia without any evidence yet of secondary osteoarthritis. I also performed the Ortolani maneuver on both of her hip joints. As in the case of Pierre, her Ortolani tests were negative, indicating no evidence of laxity or dislocation in her joints.

As I do with many patients, I referred Bronwyn to an orthopedic specialist for evaluation. Under sedation, the specialist performed a specialized procedure called a PennHIP evaluation. This special test for hip dysplasia compares joint laxity, as measured on the hip radiographs, with a range of findings for the specific breed of dog being tested. In Bronwyn's case, the PennHIP evaluation compared her joint laxity with that of other boxers.

This evaluation showed that her hips were very mildly affected. Because of the large amount of thigh and hip muscling in the boxer breed, and because of her normal PennHIP evaluation, it is unlikely that Bronwyn would ever experience problems with her hips, unlike other less muscled breeds, such as German shepherds and Labrador retrievers. In Bronwyn's case, surgery was not needed. Instead she, like Pierre, was placed on fatty acids and a supplement containing glucosamine and chondroitin.

Regarding her exercise regimen, her owner expressed concern because she wanted to show Bronwyn in dog shows and needed to train her for these shows. I suggested that she not push the dog, but rather slowly adapt her to the regimen needed for show training. By slowly working up to the required level of exercise needed, Bronwyn could best adapt to the program. If the dog was unable to work at this level due to hip pain, we would judge that based on how she acted after her workouts and adjust things accordingly.

These two cases give a good overview of how important it is to evaluate each case individually and monitor the dog's level of exercise. Making blanket recommendations is difficult, as no one can predict the future. While it is true that extra stress on the joints will cause further damage, we must remember that "dogs will be dogs." We can't keep them totally confined twenty-four hours each day. Working with your veterinarian will allow you to find the best exercise regimen for your pet.

> *Acupressure, massage, and joint-manipulation sessions, along with heat applications, which can all be done at home, are ideal forms of physical therapy that can help the arthritic pet.*

PHYSICAL THERAPY

While the physical therapy involving stretching exercises for pets is limited, you can still do things to assist your arthritic dog. Your veterinarian can show you how to do these exercises or may refer you to a physical therapist with special training in pet therapy.

Acupressure, massage, and joint-manipulation sessions, along with heat applications, which can all be done at home, are ideal forms of physical therapy that can help the arthritic pet.

Acupressure

You can be shown how to apply firm, sustained pressure to acupressure points to provide temporary relief from the pain and inflammation of arthritic joints. I often have owners do this between acupuncture treatments.

Massage

Massaging the muscles of the affected limb can help reverse the atrophy, or muscle wasting, that occurs in severely lame pets that have stopped using an arthritic limb. Muscle wasting is seen as early as three to five days after total disuse of a limb. Pets enjoy the gentle massage of the owner's hands, and the increased touching between pet and owner increases that special human-animal bond. Muscles that are massaged daily, or several times each day, regain their tone and allow the pet to use the leg more quickly once the pain and inflammation of arthritis is reversed.

Joint Manipulation

Manipulating the affected limb allows the joint to be put through its normal range of motion. Severely affected pets not using their limbs have restricted range of motion. This allows scar tissue to build up and, in severe cases, can result in permanent changes. Supervised manipulation is commonly done in pets that have undergone joint surgery, as manipulation is essential in preventing permanent lockup of the limb. Your doctor can show you how to properly and gently manipulate the pet's affected limb.

Hot Packs

Applying warmth to the sore arthritic joint can bring temporary relief to your dog. A warm water bottle or heating pad can be used to provide five to fifteen minutes of heat. Because electric heating pads can be dangerous and have resulted in severe burns in pets, it is essential that your veterinarian show you how to safely use the pad when treating your pet.

Laser Therapy

Low-level laser therapy can be used to help pets with arthritis. How exactly does laser therapy assist healing? As is true with many natural therapies, several therapeutic mechanisms have been proposed. The one most commonly accepted involves individual cells and light emission. Cells in the body emit and absorb light (biophotons) by means of chromophores (light-sensitive molecules in the cells); the light from the laser is absorbed by the chromophores and is converted to chemical energy.

These emissions and absorptions of light play key roles in regulating various cellular activities, including cell division, cell-to-cell communication, cell activation, and cell migration, all of which are essential in wound healing. Optimal results occur when the laser light is low intensity (meaning the treated tissue is not heated, unlike in laser surgery, which entails the use of lasers of a higher intensity), lasts for only a short amount of time, and pulses on and off rather than remaining static.

Laser therapy creates several effects, including increased cellular energy, reduced swelling, pain relief, muscle relaxation, and reduced inflammation. The end result of the biological interactions between the laser and the cells is healing, and the exact nature of the healing depends on the condition being treated. For example, with musculoskeletal problems, the result is a reduction of inflammation and pain.

As is true with all natural therapies, it's important to understand that laser therapy by itself is usually not the sole form of therapy. Remember that the ultimate goal is true healing, and anything that allows us to reach that goal should be used. In my practice, I combine laser therapy with other therapies (herbs, homeopathic, nutritional supplements, and so on) to offer the best chance of healing.

While laser therapy can be used to assist pets in healing from almost any medical condition, it is most commonly employed for pets with diseases of the musculoskeletal system (sprains and strains, hip dysplasia, shoulder dysplasia, elbow dysplasia, and cruciate ligament injuries, for example) and nervous system (disk disease, lumbosacral disease, and even epilepsy). The benefit of laser therapy for treating chronic arthritis in people and pets is comparable to the benefit obtained with NSAID therapy but without the side effects.

My general protocol is to use a number of supplements to allow healing and, simultaneously, to use laser therapy several times per week for three to four weeks, initially. I use the laser as needed to maintain the healing process while the pet continues a supplement regimen.

One word of caution: currently there are several laser manufacturers trying to enter the veterinary market. These manufacturers' lasers have not been thoroughly tested or approved by the FDA. Because laser therapy is considered an alternative treatment, I recommend having it done only by a holistic veterinarian with experience in a number of alternative therapies. After researching the various lasers available for treating people and pets, I chose one made by Erchonia Medical because of the large amount of research showing the benefits of therapy using this particular laser.

Here are two cases I have treated with laser therapy. Princess, a four-year-old female dachshund, had experienced an episode of intervertebral disk disease in her lower back. Steroids and muscle relaxants had been prescribed by her conventional veterinarian to immediately relieve pain and inflammation. Her owner sought my care in an attempt to decrease and ultimately stop these medications and allow Princess to return to a normal lifestyle. In addition to prescribing supplements for a maintenance protocol, I treated Princess with laser therapy twice weekly for three weeks.

I could have tried traditional acupuncture, but on her I found it easier to use laser therapy, rather than needles, at acupuncture points, as Princess did not like to sit still during her visits. Laser therapy quickly healed Princess. Each treatment lasted approximately two minutes, was painless, and was done while Princess sought comfort in her owner's arms.

The second case using laser therapy involved Natasha, a middle-aged Rottweiler who suffered lameness associated with a slight tear in her right cranial cruciate ligament. Various conventional anti-inflammatory medications did not improve her limping, and her veterinarian strongly recommended surgery. Because Natasha's owner wanted to avoid surgery if possible, she sought my care.

While surgery is necessary for some dogs with cruciate ligament injuries, in my practice I have found success in many cases by using a variety of natural remedies, thus avoiding the expensive surgery, which also requires significant postoperative rehabilitation and physical therapy. In Natasha's case, I prescribed anti-inflammatory herbs, homeopathic medicine, and joint supplements containing glucosamine and hyaluronic acid. I also treated the dog with weekly laser therapy applied to her lower back and knee. Currently, she is healing well, her lameness is decreasing, and it appears that she will be able to avoid surgery. My plan is to continue her supplement regimen indefinitely and to use laser therapy as needed to promote the healing of her damaged ligaments.

Laser therapy is not a cure-all for every pet; it is another natural therapy that has proven successful in both people and pets afflicted with various medical problems. It is inexpensive and painless, and it induces natural healing rather than the hiding of symptoms, as often occurs with conventional medications.

In pets, lasers are usually directed at acupuncture/acupressure points. The pet can be treated at the doctor's office, and in some instances an owner may be able to rent a small unit to use at home.

Electrical Stimulation

Electrical stimulation decreases pain and inflammation. It works by sending painless, harmless electrical signals that stimulate nerve endings, acting to decrease pain. Handheld units called TENS units (for "transcutaneous electrical nerve stimulation") can be purchased by owners who administer the treatment to acupuncture points designated by the veterinarian.

Ultrasound

Ultrasound uses sound waves to reduce inflammation by increasing heat and blood flow to the affected joint and surrounding tissues. The result is a warming of the area, which soothes inflamed muscles. Although popular with people, ultrasound therapy is rarely used in pets but could be a viable complementary treatment.

Exercise and physical therapy are important for pets with arthritis. Mild exercise, muscle massage, and joint manipulation allow the pet to have some normalcy in life and allow greater movement, keeping the joints functional for as long as possible. By combining a good natural diet, necessary supplements, and an intelligent exercise program, you can help your pet live a comfortable life after arthritis is diagnosed.

I've spent some time discussing exercise and dogs, but cats too need exercise. While it is harder to exercise a cat, there are some simple things you can do. The main goal is to get your cat moving, using its muscles and joints, in order to maintain good musculoskeletal health.

Consider using a laser light pen device; cats are intrigued by the focal point of light and will usually follow it when the laser is aimed at the floor. One popular laser toy is the Bolt; you can set it on automatic and it will entertain and exercise your cat for approximately fifteen minutes.

A toy that resembles a fishing pole, with the line tied to a small stuffed toy, engages many cats. They love to chase the stuffed toy as it is "fished" in front of them. Try to be creative and do what you can to get your cat moving around the house. And don't forget, whether you have a dog or a cat, work with your veterinarian to find the best and right amount of exercise that your pet can safely tolerate.

CHAPTER SUMMARY

- While few studies have been done on exercise in pets, studies in people with osteoarthritis show that exercise benefits the cardiovascular system and increases well-being.
- Let your dog set the pace in a regular exercise program.
- Swimming is a good form of exercise for the arthritic dog.
- Physical therapy enhances muscle tone to support affected joints.
- Physical therapies you can perform on your dog at home include acupressure, massage, joint manipulation, and heat application.
- Physical therapy methods that a professional can perform or train you to do include laser, electrical, and ultrasound treatments.

CHAPTER NINE

PREVENTING ARTHRITIS
in YOUR PET

I'M OFTEN ASKED IF THERE IS ANYTHING THAT CAN BE DONE to prevent arthritis in dogs and cats. While many of us like to use the word *prevent* when discussing various diseases, better terms to use may be *minimize the chance of* or *delay the onset of* the particular disease being discussed. While I believe we can do much to prevent problems such as arthritis, I hesitate to use the word *prevent* (even though I often use it with my clients or when I am being interviewed on the radio or television) because it implies something definite. In other words, if I tell you that you can prevent arthritis by following a few simple steps, this implies that your pet will never get arthritis if you follow my advice. Unfortunately, I can't make that guarantee, even though I know many of the owners who follow my advice will actually prevent arthritis in their pets.

With this in mind, here are my tips to "prevent," "minimize the chance of," or "delay the onset of " arthritis in your dog or cat.

KEEP YOUR PET LEAN. A major cause of many health issues is excess weight. As is true with people, the incidence of many chronic, inflammatory, and degenerative disorders increases as body weight increases past the ideal norm. Clinical experience confirms that pets and people who are at or slightly below their ideal weight tend to be healthier and have fewer medical problems, including arthritis. The less weight the joints need to support, especially as the joints exhibit normal wear and tear throughout the aging process, the greater the chance arthritis will be delayed or prevented.

MINIMIZE EXCESSIVE WEAR AND TEAR ON YOUR PET'S JOINTS. Dogs and cats by nature like to play and exercise. A normal amount of exercise keeps the musculoskeletal system healthy. Excessive amounts lead to excessive pressure and wear on the joints. Just how much exercise is a "safe" amount is somewhat subjective and not necessarily easy to determine.

Many of my clients show their dogs or exhibit them in agility trials. Obviously, show pets, especially those doing agility training, exercise more than the typical pet. I'm not opposed to letting pets enjoy such competition, but depending on the amount of training, there can be an excessive amount of wear on their joints. These pets, and any pets that could be considered "working pets," benefit from lifelong joint supplementation, massage, physical therapy, and hydrotherapy in an attempt to maintain joint health.

MINIMIZE YOUR PET'S EXPOSURE TO ENVIRONMENTAL TOXINS. We live in a toxic world and can't control every variable. However, there are things you can do to ensure that what goes in or on your pet's body is as natural, organic, and healthy as possible.

With that in mind, I recommend the following:

1. Minimize vaccinations. I don't know any pet whose body needs vaccines every year. Most of the vaccines we have available to us are excellent at inducing a long-lasting

immunity of five years, ten years, or even longer. While the current conventional recommendation for immunization is to administer vaccines every three years, I believe even that is too much. In my practice, I do a blood antibody test called a titer test every year and vaccinate only healthy, young pets if and when the titers indicate that vaccines may be necessary (usually every five to ten years).

2. Minimize toxins in your pet's food. Many pets are fed brand-name foods that contain animal and plant by-products and chemical additives and preservatives. These ingredients may harm your pet by causing inflammation, oxidation, and cell damage. Since there are a number of well-known natural foods available, not to mention homemade cooked or raw diets, there is no excuse for feeding your pet foods that may contribute to inflammatory conditions such as arthritis (see appendix 2 on page 191 for a list of some natural foods).

3. Minimize the use of flea and tick chemicals. Most pets I see in my practice do not need year-round neurotoxic flea and tick chemicals commonly prescribed by veterinarians. There are many safe, natural things you can do to control external parasites (such as regular bathing with any of the certified organic shampoos in the Dr. Shawn's Organics line of topical pet products). If needed, chemical flea and tick control products should be used on a limited basis to quickly kill these parasites at the same time a natural program is instituted.

REDUCE INFLAMMATION THROUGH THE USE OF REGULAR SUPPLEMENTATION. Several natural therapies that I prescribe for my patients reduce inflammation and oxidation, maintaining the health of these pets. Fish oil (omega-3 fatty acids, with both EPA and DHA) and antioxidants are very helpful.

USE JOINT SUPPLEMENTS REGULARLY. There is no question that pets suffering from arthritis should take one or more joint supplements regularly. However, all pets can benefit from regular joint supplementation.

To my knowledge, there are no controlled studies showing that starting joint supplements at an early age will prevent or delay the onset of arthritis, but it is my impression from clinical experience that this is the case. Since joint supplements tend to be free of serious side effects, there is no harm in administering these to your pet. If your pet is a working pet, I believe joint supplementation is especially helpful and should be started as soon as possible. Additionally, if your pet is a large-breed dog (these pets often experience arthritis earlier in life), joint supplementation is indicated beginning in puppyhood.

When pets are spayed or neutered in my practice, we radiograph the hip to determine the presence or absence of hip dysplasia. Pets that shows signs of hip dysplasia during this evaluation, but that do not show clinical signs and are not candidates for surgery, are placed on joint supplementation and monitored regularly for the progression of the dysplasia or the development of arthritis.

> *I recommend that all pets be radiographed when they are anesthetized for any surgical procedure in order to check for arthritis and other health problems.*

CHAPTER TEN

TYING IT ALL TOGETHER

As we come to the end of this book, I hope I've given you a better understanding of arthritis. Remember that arthritis takes months or years to evolve and that it is a painful inflammatory condition. There are other causes of lameness in pets besides arthritis, such as neurological disorders and cancers. *A proper diagnosis is essential before choosing any therapy.*

Conventional medications, such as corticosteroids and nonsteroidal anti-inflammatory medications, do have their place in the treatment of some arthritic pets, but these drugs can result in detrimental side effects, which makes using them as the sole long-term therapy a poor choice for any but the very few pets that do not improve with any other treatment. When they are necessary, conventional medications should be used in a holistic fashion: the lowest dose that provides relief to pets should be used as infrequently as possible to avoid serious side effects.

Natural therapies all have their place in the treatment of pets with arthritis. Often one of them can serve as the sole therapy. When needed, lower doses of conventional medications can be combined with natural remedies to help pets on extremely painful days.

Here, then, is my approach to arthritic pets:

1. First, a correct diagnosis is important. And because arthritis is a degenerative process, the earlier a correct diagnosis is made and the proper treatment is started, the sooner we can attempt to make pets feel better and slow down the destruction of the joint.

2. Once we can pinpoint the location of the lameness or pain and are comfortable that we are not dealing with some other cause of lameness (immunological joint destruction, infectious arthritis, neurological disease, or cancer), we perform diagnostic testing. This usually involves taking radiographs (X-rays) of the affected bones and joints. Because of the different views that must be obtained in order to fully evaluate the joints and because many arthritic pets are in pain, the radiographs are usually taken while pets are under heavy sedation or anesthesia.

3. Ancillary diagnostic testing, such as blood and urine testing, may be needed to make sure that internal diseases are not causing the clinical signs. Also, since many pets are older animals, it's important to diagnose and treat any co-existing conditions. And if drug therapy, such as nonsteroidal medications, must be given, it is important to make sure that any underlying problems that could worsen with conventional medicines, such as kidney or liver disease, are not present.

4. After I make my diagnosis, I discuss the numerous treatment options with the owners. I often treat pets in severe pain with traditional medical therapy, such as low doses

of nonsteroidal medications, over a short time to give quick relief. And I place most if not all pets on oral joint supplements, herbs, and homotoxicology medications. Pets with severely debilitating arthritis may be started on weekly injections of chondroprotective agents to achieve a faster result while waiting for the oral supplements to kick in.

5. Laser therapy, acupuncture, and/or chiropractic therapy are used as needed. Typically, I use laser therapy treatments twice weekly for one month and then as needed to maintain the pets' healing process. Laser therapy can produce fast and dramatic results and is not painful for pets or expensive for owners.

Each doctor develops his or her favorite approach to dealing with various disorders, including arthritis. In order to treat pets holistically, it's important to do what's best for the pets' overall health and well-being. Pets must be treated humanely. Owners should be involved in treatment decisions for their pets.

There is no hard and fast rule I use when deciding what treatment is best for particular patients. I explain options to the owners, including side effects and costs of the treatments. The owners and I form a team whose goal it is to do what's best for the pets. When owners are involved, they are more likely to take an interest in the therapy. They are vital members of the treatment team and know they are important to the pets' outcome. This is a far different approach from that of the doctor who sees himself or herself as "God" and uses "shotgun" therapy with no owner involvement. Owners are loving, dedicated, kindhearted people. It is essential that they be involved in the decision-making process, as they are ultimately responsible for their pets.

For more information about holistic pet care, or to find a holistic veterinarian in your area, contact the American Holistic

Veterinary Medical Association at 410-569-0795 and visit the Pet Care Naturally website at www.petcarenaturally.com.

Owners should be involved in treatment decisions for their pets.

ACKNOWLEDGMENTS

Thanks to all my clients, who trust me with their pets.

Thanks to all my wonderful patients, who give me the chance to heal them in a natural, organic way, rather than to simply make them feel better by covering up their pain with numerous medications.

Thanks to my beautiful wife and daughter for your encouragement and support.

Thanks to God for giving me the gift of holistic care and the ability to share this gift with you.

Thanks to all my colleagues who refer their challenging and difficult cases to my hospital.

Thanks to my colleagues in the American Holistic Veterinary Medical Association for sharing your knowledge and passion with me.

Thanks to all those who allow me to educate others by speaking at their events, club meetings, and veterinary conferences.

Thanks to all of you who have guided me over the years. There are too many to name, but you know who you are and how much you mean to me. Your guidance and wisdom have helped save the lives of numerous pets and provided untold years of pleasure for their owners.

RESULTS *of a* CLINICAL TRIAL USING TWO NOVEL HA SUPPLEMENTS *in* DOGS

OSTEOARTHRITIS IS THE MOST COMMON CAUSE of skeletal disease and lameness in older dogs and cats. Most older pets, especially large breed dogs, will develop osteoarthritis in one or more joints. Typically, the joints that will be affected include the thoracic and lumbar vertebrae, hips, and knees. In cats, joints of the small bones of the front and back feet may also be affected.

Conventional therapies for the treatment of osteoarthritis are aimed at reducing pain and inflammation, which in turn decreases lameness and increases range of motion of the affected joints. Corticosteroids, such as prednisone, and nonsteroidal anti-inflammatory medications (NSAIDs) are commonly prescribed, and NSAIDs are among the most prescribed medications for pets and people with osteoarthritis. While effective, the conventional medications cause a number of side effects, including further damage to the joint cartilage, liver disease, kidney disease, gastrointestinal disease, weight gain, diabetes, adrenal gland disorders, and osteoporosis.

In a search to find a safer, more natural alternative to treat osteoarthritis, a number of companies have successfully marketed various joint supplements. These include glucosamine, chondroitin, shark cartilage, MSM, perna, and various anti-inflammatory herbs. Recently, two new joint supplements containing hyaluronic acid (hyaluronan, HA) have been developed and released to the veterinary community. Here are the results of clinical testing of these supplements.

The two products tested were Glycovet (now called Cholo Gel) and Cholodin Flex, available through MVP Laboratories in Omaha, Nebraska. Cholo Gel is a viscous gel, and Cholodin Flex is a flavored, chewable pill/treat. Cholo Gel is a multiplex of very specific oligomers of hyaluronan, which are absorbed through the mucous membranes of the mouth. The longer the pet can retain the liquid in the mouth, the better the results. This is why it is suggested that the gel be put on food or a treat. The hyaluronan in the products comes from the fermentation of a bacterium that secretes the hyaluronan into the media.

The proposed mechanisms of action for hyaluronan are as follows.

First, HA reduces swelling at the site of injury by decreasing leukocyte transmigration and infiltration into the affected tissue. It does this by binding to the CD44 binding sites on the leukocytes. If there is enough hyaluronan available to bind to the CD44 sites on the leukocytes, fewer leukocytes will reach the area of trauma, resulting in reduced swelling and pain.

Second, HA inhibits the arachidonic acid pathway (similar to the anti-inflammatory actions of corticosteroids and NSAIDs). Bradykinin is produced by serine proteases (tissue kallikreins) cleaving high- and low-molecular-weight kininogens. Hyaluronan blocks the serine protease activity so that lysyl bradykinin, bradykinin, and arachidonic acid cannot be produced, resulting in decreased inflammation and pain.

Research subjects were obtained via a weekly newspaper column soliciting owners of dogs with arthritis. Before entering the four-week study, the dogs were given physical examinations to rule out neurological disease. In some cases, previous radiographs (X-rays) were evaluated to assess cartilage damage. In many cases, no previous radiographs were available. These patients' diagnosis of osteoarthritis was based on history, clinical signs, ruling out other causes of lameness, and prior response to either corticosteroids or NSAIDs. Some dogs were at the time taking NSAIDs or another joint supplement. If the patient response to the NSAIDs or joint supplements was excellent (the patient's lameness was 100 percent better), the pet was taken off the NSAIDs or joint supplements at the start of the study in order to properly assess the product being tested. If the response was less than 100 percent (the owner stated that the pet still exhibited lameness), the medication or other supplement was continued and Cholo Gel or Cholodin Flex was administered; the pet was monitored to see if the residual lameness improved even further (100 percent response) on the new supplement.

Pets were chosen to receive either Cholo Gel or Cholodin Flex chewable tablets. Older dogs exhibiting any signs of cognitive disorder were administered the tablets (which contain choline, a compound that has been shown to improve signs of cognitive disorder); the other participants were administered the gel, which contains only the HA without choline. Thirteen dogs received the gel and thirty-nine received the tablets. The initial dose of the gel was three to five drops twice daily regardless of weight. The tablets were dosed at one-half tablet twice daily for dogs weighing 25 pounds and less, and one tablet twice daily for dogs weighing more than 25 pounds. Owners were instructed to double the dose of the gel or the tablet after two weeks if no improvement was noted.

Following the four-week trial, owners were contacted by telephone and asked the following four questions:

1. What previous course of therapy had been used, and how effective was the therapy?
2. In your opinion, was this case mild, moderate/routine, or severe?
3. How would you rate your pet's improvement with this new supplement: excellent, very good, good, moderate, slight, or no change?
4. Would you use this supplement again?

The results of the study are as follows:

For pets taking the gel formulation (Cholo Gel), all owners questioned would use the supplement again. Three pets were judged by the owners to have severe disease, and seven pets were judged to have moderate or routine disease. Three owners did not respond to follow-up phone calls. Pets' response to the gel was considered moderate by four owners, good by five owners, and excellent by one owner. Interestingly, several owners indicated that their pets experienced only a poor to fair response to prior therapy with NSAID administration, which is the most common therapy for pets with arthritis.

For pets taking the chewable tablet (Cholodin Flex), which also contains choline, four owners said they would not use the supplement again, as they saw no response to the therapy. Fourteen pets were judged by the owners to have severe disease, two pets were judged to have mild disease, and ten pets were judged to have moderate or routine disease. Thirteen owners did not respond to follow-up phone calls. Response to Cholodin Flex was considered slight by four owners, moderate by four owners, good by three owners, very good by six owners, and excellent by five owners. As with the administration of the gel, several owners indicated that the pets experienced only poor to fair response to prior therapy with NSAID administration.

Based on owner observation, it appears that administration of either the Cholo Gel or Cholodin Flex chewable tablets was effective in controlling symptoms of lameness and pain seen in dogs with osteoarthritis. The overall rate of success for both products based on owner response to follow-up phone calls was 77 percent (success defined as at least a moderate improvement in the dog's symptoms compared to either no treatment or other therapy prior to starting the supplement).

As the clinical testing revealed, both the Cholo Gel and Cholodin Flex were effective in treating osteoarthritis in dogs. Either product is a suitable, safe alternative to the use of corticosteroids or NSAIDs in the treatment of this common, chronic, and disabling condition.

In my own practice, I have seen even more dramatic results when using either of these two products. This is likely due to the following reasons: earlier diagnosis of arthritis in my patients; coadministration of other supplements, such as fish oil, antioxidants, and homotoxicology medications; and cotreatment with laser therapy or acupuncture. I have had particularly good results when using Cholo Gel in dogs with moderate to severe arthritis that have not shown a positive response to other joint supplements.

NATURAL PET FOODS

THE FOLLOWING BRANDS are among some of the more commonly prescribed natural pet foods. Inclusion in this list does not indicate endorsement or recommendation. Likewise, exclusion does not indicate a product is unacceptable. New products are introduced regularly, and your veterinarian can guide you in choosing the best food for your pet.

Acana	Nature's Variety
Addiction	Orijen
Blue	Solid Gold
Canidae	Taste of the Wild
EVO	Trilogy
Holistic Select	Wellness
Innova	Wysong
Natural Balance	

SOME *of* DR. SHAWN'S FAVORITE JOINT PRODUCTS

MANY DIFFERENT PRODUCTS ON THE MARKET can be highly beneficial for the dog or cat with arthritis. I've listed just a few of the products I like and prescribe for my patients.

JOINT SUPPLEMENTS

Adequan, by Novartis
Cholo Gel/Cholodin Flex, by MVP Laboratories
Cosequin, by Nutramax Laboratories
Glyco-Flex, by Vetri-Science Laboratories
MegaFlex, by Rx Vitamins for Pets
ProMotion, by Animal Health Options

ANTIOXIDANTS

Proanthozone, by Animal Health Options
Rx Essentials, by Rx Vitamins for Pets

FATTY ACIDS

Ultra EFA, by Rx Vitamins for Pets

MISCELLANEOUS PRODUCTS

Vetri-DMG, by Vetri-Science Laboratories

Vim & Vigor, a health maintenance formula made by Pet-Togethers

BIBLIOGRAPHY

Ackerman, L. "Dermatologic Uses of Fatty Acids in Dogs and Cats." *Veterinary Medicine* (December 1995): 1149–1155.

———. "Nondermatologic Indications for Fatty Acid Supplementation in Dogs and Cats." *Veterinary Medicine* (December 1995): 1156–1159.

———. "Reviewing the Biochemical Properties of Fatty Acids." *Veterinary Medicine* (December 1995): 1138–1148.

Altman S. "Small Animal Acupuncture: Scientific Basis and Clinical Applications." In *Complementary and Alternative Veterinary Medicine: Principles and Practice*, ed. A. Schoen and S. Wynn, 147–168. St. Louis, MO: Mosby, 1998.

Anderson, M. A., M. R. Slater, and T. A. Hammad. "Results of a Survey of Small Animal Practitioners on the Perceived Clinical Efficacy and Safety of an Oral Nutraceutical." *Preventive Veterinary Medicine* 38 (1999): 65–73.

Balch, J., and P. Balch. *Prescription for Nutritional Healing*. New York: Avery Publishing, 1997.

Bardet, J. F. "Lameness." In *Textbook of Veterinary Internal Medicine*. 4th ed., ed. S. Ettinger and E. Feldman, 136–143. Philadelphia: W. B. Saunders, 1995.

Belfield, W. "Orthomolecular Medicine: A Practitioner's Perspective." In *Complementary and Alternative Veterinary Medicine: Principles and Practice*, ed. A. Schoen and S. Wynn, 113–132. St. Louis, MO: Mosby, 1998.

Bennet, D. "Treatment of the Immune-Mediated Inflammatory Arthropathies of the Dog and Cat." In *Kirk's Current Veterinary Therapy XII*, ed. J. Bonagura, 1188–1195. Philadelphia: W. B. Saunders, 1995.

Bennett, D., and C. May. "Joint Diseases of Dogs and Cats." In *Textbook of Veterinary Internal Medicine*. 4th ed., ed. S. Ettinger and E. Feldman, 2032–2077. Philadelphia: W. B. Saunders, 1995.

Beren, J. J., S. L. Hill, and N. R. Rose. "Therapeutic Effects of Cosamin® on Autoimmune Type II Collagen Induced Arthritis in Rats." Paper presented to the 1997 North American Veterinary Conference, Orlando, Florida.

Bratman, S., and D. Kroll. *Natural Health Bible*. Rocklin, CA: Prima Publishing, 1999.

Chen, J. *Clinical Manual of Oriental Medicine*, 54–59, 551–562. City of Industry, CA: Lotus Herbs, 1999.

D'Ambrosia, E., B. Casa, G. Bompani et al. "Glucosamine Sulfate: A Controlled Clinical Evaluation in Arthrosis." *Pharmatherapeutica* (1981): 2, 504.

Day, C. *The Homeopathic Treatment of Small Animals*. London: C. W. Daniel Essex, 1990.

Day, C., and J. G. G. Saxton. "Veterinary Homeopathy: Principles and Practice." In *Complementary and Alternative Veterinary Medicine: Principles and Practice*, ed. A. Schoen and S. Wynn, 485–514. St. Louis, MO: Mosby, 1998.

DeCava, J. "Glandular Supplements." *Nutrition News and Views* (West Barnstable, MA) (May–June 1997).

de Guzman, E. "Western Herbal Medicine: Clinical Applications." In *Complementary and Alternative Veterinary Medicine: Principles and Practice*, ed. A. Schoen and S. Wynn, 337–378. St. Louis, MO: Mosby, 1998.

Fox, S. M., and S. Campbell. "Update: Two Years (1997–1998) Clinical Experience with Rimadyl (carprofen) August, 1999.

Frost, M. *Going Back to the Basics*. San Diego: privately published by M. Frost, 1997.

Grazi, S., and M. Costa. *SAMe (S-adenosylmethionine)*, 1–14, 31–46, 60–78, 79–98, 211–224. Rocklin, CA: Prima Publishing, 1999.

Hobbs, R., and G. Bucco. *The Natural Pharmacist: Everything You Need to Know about Arthritis.* Rocklin, CA: Prima Publishing, 1999.

Hudson, Donald, and Doreen Hudson. "Magnetic Field Therapy." In *Complementary and Alternative Veterinary Medicine: Principles and Practice,* ed. A. Schoen and S. Wynn, 75–296. St. Louis, MO: Mosby, 1998.

Hulse, D. S., D. Hart, M. Slatter, and B. S. Beale. "The Effect of Cosequin in Cranial Cruciate Deficient and Reconstructed Stifle Joints in Dogs." Paper presented to the Veterinary Orthopedic Society, 25th Annual Conference, February 1998: 64.

Johnson, K. "Treatment of Osteomyelitis, Discospondylitis, and Septic Arthritis." In *Kirk's Current Veterinary Therapy XII,* ed. J. Bonagura, 1200–1204. Philadelphia: W. B. Saunders, 1995.

Johnson, K., and A. D. J. Watson. "Skeletal Diseases." In *Textbook of Veterinary Internal Medicine.* 5th ed., ed. S. Ettinger and E. Feldman, 1887–1916. Philadelphia: W. B. Saunders, 2000.

Johnson, K., A. D. J. Watson, and R. Page. "Skeletal Diseases." In *Textbook of Veterinary Internal Medicine.* 4th ed., ed. S. Ettinger and E. Feldman, 2077–2103. Philadelphia: W. B. Saunders, 1995.

Kandel, J., and D. Sudderth. *The Arthritis Solution.* Rocklin, CA: Prima Publishing, 1997.

Kendall, R. "Therapeutic Nutrition for the Cat, Dog, and Horse." In *Complementary and Alternative Veterinary Medicine: Principles and Practice,* ed. A. Schoen and S. Wynn, 53–72. St. Louis, MO: Mosby, 1998.

Lane, I. W. "Shark Cartilage: Its Potential Medical Applications." *Journal of Advancement in Medicine* 4, no. 4 (1991): 263–271.

Lane, I. W., and L. Comac. *Sharks Don't Get Cancer.* New York: Avery, 1993.

Lane, I. W., and E. Contreras Jr. "High Rate of Bioactivity (Reduction in Gross Tumor Size) Observed in Advanced Cancer Patients Treated with Shark Cartilage Material." *Journal of Naturopathic Medicine* 31 (1992): 86–88.

Lees, P. "Inflammation and the Pharmacology of Anti-inflammatory Drugs." In *New Advances in Control of Pain and Inflammation, Proceedings of the Academy of Veterinary Internal Medicine,* 7–20. N.p.: Academy of Veterinary Internal Medicine, 1997.

Lewis, L., M. Morris Jr., and M. Hand. *Small Animal Clinical Nutrition.* 3rd ed., 31–33, 41–42, 61–63. Topeka, KS: Mark Morris Associates, 1987.

Lopes, A. "Double-Blind Clinical Evaluation of the Relative Efficacy of Ibuprofen and Glucosamine Sulphate in the Management of Osteoarthrosis of the Knee in Outpatients." *Current Medical Research & Opinion* 8 (1982): 145.

Macleod, G. *Dogs: Homeopathic Remedies.* Essex, U.K.: C. W. Daniel, 1992.

Magne, M. "Swollen Joints and Lameness." In *Textbook of Veterinary Internal Medicine.* 5th ed., ed. S. Ettinger and E. Feldman, 77–79. Philadelphia: W. B. Saunders, 2000.

Manley, P. "The Treatment of Degenerative Joint Disease." In *Kirk's Current Veterinary Therapy XII*, ed. J. Bonagura, 1196–1199. Philadelphia: W. B. Saunders, 1995.

Matz, M. "Gastrointestinal Ulcer Therapy." In *Kirk's Current Veterinary Therapy XII*, ed. J. Bonagura 706–710. Philadelphia: W. B. Saunders, 1995.

McDonald, R., and V. Langston. "Use of Corticosteroids and Non-steroidal Anti-inflammatory Agents." In *Textbook of Veterinary Internal Medicine.* 4th ed., ed. S. Ettinger and E. Feldman, 284–293. Philadelphia: W. B. Saunders, 1995.

McNamara, P., S. Barr, and H. Erb. "Hematologic, Hemostatic, and Biochemical Effects in Dogs Receiving an Oral Chondroprotective Agent for Thirty Days." *American Journal of Veterinary Research* 57, no. 9 (September 1996): 1390–1394.

Moore, K. "LLT for the Treatment of Chronic Pain." *Frontiers in Electro-Optics, Conference Proceedings* (1990): 283–290.

Morrison, R. "Magnetic Healing." *Dog and Kennel* (October 1999): 36–38.

Murray, M. *The Healing Power of Herbs*, 378–379. Rocklin, CA: Prima Publishing, 1995.

Murray, M., and J. Pizzorno. *Encyclopedia of Natural Medicine.* 2nd ed. Rocklin, CA: Prima Publishing, 1998.

Murray, R. *Natural vs. Synthetic, Life vs. Death, Truth vs. the Lie.* Palmyra, WI: Standard Process, 1995.

Papich, M., and E. Hardie. "Management of Chronic Pain." In *New Advances in Control of Pain and Inflammation, Proceedings of the Academy of Veterinary Internal Medicine*, 61–70. N.p.: Academy of Veterinary Internal Medicine, 1997.

Pedersen, N., H. Morgan, and P. Vasseur. "Joint Diseases of Dogs and Cats." In *Textbook of Veterinary Internal Medicine.* 5th ed., ed. S. Ettinger and E. Feldman, 1862–1886. Philadelphia: W. B. Saunders, 2000.

Pfizer Animal Health Technical Bulletin. "First-Year Clinical Experience with Rimadyl (carprofen): Assessment of Product Safety, May 1998."

Philippi, A., C. Leffler, and S. Leffler. "Glucosamine, Chondroitin, and Manganese Ascorbate for Degenerative Joint Disease of the Knee or Low Back: A Randomized Double-Blind Placebo-Controlled Study." *Military Medicine* 164 (February 1999): 85–91.

Pitcairn, R., and S. Pitcairn. *Dr. Pitcairn's Complete Guide to Natural Health for Dogs and Cats,* 235–236. Emmaus, PA: Rodale, 1995.

Plumb, D. *Veterinary Drug Handbook.* 3rd ed., 102–103, 260–261, 306–308, 528–535. Ames: Iowa State University Press, 1999.

Richardson, D. "Developmental Orthopedics: Nutritional Influences in the Dog." In *Textbook of Veterinary Internal Medicine.* 4th ed., ed. S. Ettinger and E. Feldman, 252–257. Philadelphia: W. B. Saunders, 1995.

Rosenfeld, I. *Dr. Rosenfeld's Guide to Alternative Medicine,* 208–216. New York: Random House, 1996.

Schoen, A. M. "Acupuncture for Musculoskeletal Disorders." In *Veterinary Acupuncture,* ed. A. Schoen. St. Louis, MO: Mosby, 1994.

Schrader, S. "Differential Diagnosis of Nontraumatic Causes of Lameness in Young Growing Dogs." In *Kirk's Current Veterinary Therapy XII,* ed. J. Bonagura, 1171–1180. Philadelphia: W. B. Saunders, 1995.

———. "The Use of the Laboratory in the Diagnosis of Joint Disorders of Dogs and Cats." In *Kirk's Current Veterinary Therapy XII,* ed. J. Bonagura, 1166–1171. Philadelphia: W. B. Saunders, 1995.

Schwartz, C. "Chinese Herbal Medicine in Small Animal Practice." In *Complementary and Alternative Veterinary Medicine: Principles and Practice,* ed. A. Schoen and S. Wynn, 437–450. St. Louis, MO: Mosby, 1998.

Smith, G., and P. McKelvie. "Current Concepts in the Diagnosis of Canine Hip Dysplasia." In *Kirk's Current Veterinary Therapy XII,* ed. J. Bonagura, 1180–1188. Philadelphia: W. B. Saunders, 1995.

Strazza, M. "Magnetic Field Exposure as an Adjunct Therapeutic Modality in the Dog, Cat, and Horse." In *Journal of the American Holistic Veterinary Medical Association* 15, no. 2 (May–July 1996): 27–31.

Strombeck, D. *Home-Prepared Dog and Cat Diets,* 217–236. Ames: Iowa State University Press, 1999.

Thompson, J. "Immunologic Diseases." In *Textbook of Veterinary Internal Medicine.* 4th ed., ed. S. Ettinger and E. Feldman, 2002–2029. Philadelphia: W. B. Saunders, 1995.

Tilford, G., and M. Wulff-Tilford. *All You Ever Wanted to Know about Herbs for Pets*, 66–68, 170–173, 264–269. Irvine, CA: BowTie Press, 1999.

Ullman, D. "Homeopathic Medicine: Principles and Research." In *Complementary and Alternative Veterinary Medicine: Principles and Practice*, ed. A. Schoen and S. Wynn, 469–484. St. Louis, MO: Mosby, 1998.

Whitaker, J. *Dr. Whitaker's Guide to Natural Healing*, 163, 310. Rocklin, CA: Prima Publishing, 1996.

Wilson, J. "Shark Cartilage: A Review of Background Literature and Research." *Townsend Letter for Doctors* (August–September 1994).

Wolfsheimer, K. "Obesity." In *Textbook of Veterinary Internal Medicine*. 5th ed., ed. S. Ettinger and E. Feldman, 70–71. Philadelphia: W. B. Saunders, 2000.

INDEX

ABOUT *the* AUTHOR

DR. SHAWN MESSONNIER is a well-known holistic veterinarian and pet care advocate. He graduated in 1987 from Texas A&M University with a Doctorate of Veterinary Medicine. In 1991, he opened Paws & Claws Animal Hospital, the first referral hospital for dogs, cats, and exotic pets in Plano, Texas.

After using conventional therapies for several years, Dr. Shawn became convinced that many of the pets that were not improving with lifelong use of conventional medications might respond better to alternative treatments. This desire to improve the quality of his patients' lives led him to become adept at treating pets with a variety of natural treatments. Because of his success with these therapies, Dr. Shawn created the Acupuncture and Holistic Animal Health Care Center, the only hospital in the Plano area to offer both conventional and natural therapies for dogs and cats.

Dr. Shawn is the author of a number of books, including the award-winning *Natural Health Bible for Dogs & Cats* and *Unexpected*

Miracles: Hope and Holistic Healing for Pets, as well as *The Natural Vet's Guide to Preventing and Treating Cancer in Dogs*, *8 Weeks to a Healthy Dog*, and *The Allergy Solution for Dogs*.

Dr. Shawn regularly writes articles and columns for several prestigious publications, including *Dog Fancy*, *Dog World*, *Fido Friendly*, *Natural Awakenings*, *Whole Living*, and *Animal Wellness*.

He is the holistic veterinary consultant for Pet-Togethers (www.pettogethers.net/healthypet), a leading manufacturer of natural pet care products.

Each week, pet owners around the world listen to his award-winning radio show, *Dr. Shawn, The Natural Vet*, on the Martha Stewart Living channel on SiriusXM Satellite Radio.

His website, www.petcarenaturally.com, has also won awards and continues to be the number one website on natural pet care.

Dr. Shawn has developed the only application for the iPhone on the topic of natural pet care. His unique line of certified organic pet shampoos and his herbal ear wash (Dr. Shawn's Organics) continue to be highly praised by pet owners around the world. They are the only topical products that have been proven both effective and safe for frequent use.

Dr. Shawn is also a speaker and consultant. His popular lectures teach veterinarians and pet owners how holistic approaches can reduce the cost of veterinary care and help pets live longer, healthier lives. His lecture style is unique, often combining humor and magic to enforce his message. He challenges those he works with to be the best they can be, to rise above any challenges they may face. He is committed to providing the best health care for his patients.

Dr. Shawn regularly consults with pet owners around the world to help them choose the most holistic pet therapies.

Contact Dr. Messonnier about speaking and consulting at:

2145 West Park Blvd.
Plano, TX 75075

Phone: 972-867-8800

Email: naturalvet@juno.com
Website: www.petcarenaturally.com

NEW WORLD LIBRARY is dedicated to publishing books and other media that inspire and challenge us to improve the quality of our lives and the world.

We are a socially and environmentally aware company, and we strive to embody the ideals presented in our publications. We recognize that we have an ethical responsibility to our customers, our staff members, and our planet.

We serve our customers by creating the finest publications possible on personal growth, creativity, spirituality, wellness, and other areas of emerging importance. We serve New World Library employees with generous benefits, significant profit sharing, and constant encouragement to pursue their most expansive dreams.

As a member of the Green Press Initiative, we print an increasing number of books with soy-based ink on 100 percent postconsumer-waste recycled paper. Also, we power our offices with solar energy and contribute to nonprofit organizations working to make the world a better place for us all.

Our products are available
in bookstores everywhere.
For our catalog, please contact:

New World Library
14 Pamaron Way
Novato, California 94949

Phone: 415-884-2100 or 800-972-6657
Catalog requests: Ext. 50
Orders: Ext. 52
Fax: 415-884-2199
Email: escort@newworldlibrary.com

To subscribe to our electronic newsletter, visit
www.newworldlibrary.com